Self Observation:
The Awakening of Conscience

D0954803

Self Observation:
The Awakening of Conscience

10/09

An Owner's Manual

*for my old friend & fellow teacher whose example of
courage & integrity is an inspiration to me —
w/love & Respect*

Red Hawk

Red Hawk

"Know Thyself."

HOHM PRESS
Prescott, Arizona

© 2009, Robert Moore

All rights reserved. No part of this book may be reproduced in any manner without written permission from the publisher, except in the case of quotes used in critical articles and reviews.

Cover design: Zac Parker, Kadak Graphics, Prescott, Arizona

Interior design and layout: Kubera Book Design, Prescott, Arizona

Library of Congress Cataloging-in-Publication Data

Red Hawk.
  Self observation : the awakening of conscience : an owner's manual / Red Hawk.
    p. cm.
  Includes bibliographical references and index.
  ISBN 978-1-890772-92-5 (trade pbk. : alk. paper)
  1. Observation (Psychology) 2. Introspection.
  BF76.6.O27R44 2009
  158.1--dc22
                                2008056157

HOHM PRESS
P.O. Box 2501
Prescott, AZ 86302
800-381-2700
http://www.hohmpress.com

This book was printed in the U.S.A. on recycled, acid-free paper using soy ink.

Dedication

For Yogi Ramsuratkumar: Source

For Mister Lee: Inspiration, Outlaw Saint, True Friend

For Andre Enard: Information about the crucial function of sensation in self observation; Teacher of Dancing

For Maxie: Feeling and feedback

For Rain Drop & Little Wind: Reasons to begin

For Iain, Jett & Jayce: Reasons to continue

For Regina Sara Ryan: Great help in editing

Contents

CHAPTER 1

Self Observation—Know Thyself

Knowing others is wisdom;
Knowing the self is enlightenment.
(Lao Tsu. *Tao Te Ching*, Sutra 33)

Know Thyself, weary Traveler.

I am lost. I have forgotten who I am and why I came here.

Know Thyself is one of the foundational spiritual teachings of humanity. It has been taught by masters as long as there have been humans as we know them, that is with a neo-cortex or human brain. It was written over the gate to Pythagoras' School. It was above the entrance to the Oracle at Delphi. Socrates taught it to his students, Krishna, Buddha, Lao Tsu, Jesus, Rama, they all taught it. On the path of awakening, this teaching is fundamental.

And the essential tool to Know Thyself is simple self observation. Buddha calls it watching. Krishna calls it meditation. Jesus calls it witnessing. Mister Gurdjieff calls it self observation. It is a form of prayer without words. It is meditation in action. Unless and until I come to know myself, I am driven by habits which I do not see and over which I have no control; I am a machine, an automaton, a robot moving in circles, constantly repeating myself.

I am not aware, but unconscious, habitual, *mechanical.**[1] I imagine I am conscious, awake, aware because my eyes are open. But habit is unconscious, automatic-pilot, without volition or *intention**; inside I am asleep.

What is more, because I am unconscious, a creature of habit, I do harm to myself, my relationships, and my environment. The human body is mammal; all mammals are creatures of habit. We are herd animals. This is a very powerful force in the body, impossible to ignore; it causes me to lose the thread of who I am = *attention** (*consciousness**) and identify myself as the body, so powerful is the need to identify with, and be included as, part of the herd. Herd animals do not think for themselves, the herd thinks for them and acts for them. Whatever direction the herd goes in, we go. Even if we are led over a cliff, we will follow to our death rather than go against the herd and think for ourselves. To think for myself, to know myself, risks being expelled from the herd, a death-sentence for a mammal. Security is the herd. An isolated grazer away from the herd is dead meat, easy prey for predators. Deep in our instinct, all of us know this and fear being isolated from the herd. So to get a mammal to think for herself, to observe herself, to know herself, is very difficult. It is not natural to mammal behavior. It requires conscious effort and intent. It requires courage and *will of attention.** As far as I can tell, humans are the only mammals who have the capability of observing themselves.

I am not suggesting that if I come to know myself my habits will change. They have a lifetime of momentum and emotional force. They repeat. What can change in me is my relationship to this body of habits. This is called a "shift in context." As I am now,

---

[1]　Words marked with a star and italicized the first time they are used are defined in the Glossary at the end of this book.

I am identified (= "I am that") with my habits. I identify myself *as* my habits, they are who I am. Thus, "I" and the habits are one, the same. I am identified. With patient, honest, steady, sincere self observation this *identification** can shift. I can begin to view the habit *objectively,** that is without identification, as a scientist views a bug under a microscope. This is struggle with habit, not against; observation will show me what to struggle with and how to struggle. P.D. Ouspensky cites the exception to struggling against habit as the struggle against expressing *negative emotion**; this does not create unexpected or undesirable consequences (*In Search of the Miraculous.* New York: Harcourt, 1946. 12). I can begin to study the mammal body and learn its habits. Because it is a creature of habit, it repeats and I can begin to discern its patterns, intellectual, emotional, and physical. I can come to know myself.

The body is a mammal instrument, a creature of habit. Thus, it is predictable. The doe follows the exact same path to the water hole every day. The lion observes this and learns to wait on a low-lying limb for her to come down the path. In the same way, the inner observer can begin to predict the habitual behavior of the mammal instrument, the body, and be prepared for it. It learns the patterns. It knows itself. This is my only hope for becoming more conscious and not at the mercy of habit; if I see the habit often enough, say 10,000 times or more, then I can begin to predict where, when, and how it will manifest exactly as it has so many times before, and I may be prepared before it arises. I may be able to choose another course. Certainly I may be able to view the habit more objectively. In this way, I can cease to be always a victim of my own habits. I can begin to find some stability within, some equilibrium, some moderation of tone, behavior, emotion and thought. I can recover natural sanity and *"basic goodness."**

Self observation is the tool by which this is possible. It is called "the first tool" by some, and by others "the human tool." It is the tool by which the human is able to operate, repair, and maintain the human body, tame and train its functions. Without it, I am a machine, an automaton, a robot at the mercy of unconscious, habitual, mechanical forces, both internal and external. Self observation is fundamental to the process of the *soul's** awakening from its unconscious dreaming. Thus, even an idiot can learn to operate the *instrument** (*see* human biological instrument) effectively and efficiently by learning to use the tool which comes with the instrument. To become efficient in the use of the tool requires practice. The practice is self observation. I am a mechanic; I have learned some things about how to use the tool which comes with the instrument. I am no master, but I am a good mechanic because I have developed attention to the instrument. We all know that a good mechanic, one who is honest, efficient, practical, and aware, can be of great service. This is an owner's manual written by a mechanic.

In the beginning it is good and responsible to note this important word of caution: what is being discussed here is not a *way of faith*, it is a way of self-study, of self-knowledge, a way to Know Thyself. Therefore, nothing here should be taken on faith; everything here should be, *must* be verified by your own personal experience. I am no master, merely a good mechanic. Safety lies in no longer taking the word of others for anything. Too long we have followed blindly, like sheep, like herd animals following the leader, even when the leader leads the herd over a cliff or into war.

Everything must be verified by personal experience, otherwise it is merely another form of slavery, one more chain to bind me in my unconscious and mechanical slavery. Verify, verify, verify everything for yourself. Free yourself of the habits of a lifetime, of blind following, of not thinking for yourself. There is no better or safer path to freedom.

I repeat, what we are practicing here is not a way of faith. That is a different way altogether. However, it does not mean there is not room for faith on this path; certainly there is. In fact, what one finds as she engages this "practical work on self" over a long enough period of time is this: if she began with faith, her faith is strengthened by understanding gained from self observation without judgment; if she began with no faith—as I did—then she will find that she has gained faith. So you see the wonderful irony of it? This is not a faith-based path, because faith is a gift of grace; it comes from the *Creator** to those in need of it. By our own efforts we cannot gain faith. However, by our own efforts we can *prepare the soil to receive faith*. That is one of the many rewards of the *Work*.* Here we must accept nothing on faith; we are asked to verify everything, everything, for ourselves as to its merits, its truth or falsity. We do so via patient self observation without judgment and via our personal experience.

Know Thyself

Socrates exhorted His disciples to do so;
every Master including Jesus, who called it witnessing,
has taught his disciples to observe themselves,

so they might come to know themselves. On the other hand,
I am no Master and I say, Don't do it for God's sake!
They never tell us the terrible trouble it brings,

how we will never sleep easily again
in our unconscious selfish mad habits, how
what is now unconscious, hidden in us

will be revealed, like
opening a locked cellar door, turning on
the light and what you find down there

is the county asylum crawling with inmates,
some wrapped in torn filthy sheets, others
naked and drooling; they are clawing and scratching

to gain position on the stairs, to escape, and
standing calmly in their midst, dressed
in robes of Light, is an Angel around whom

most of them huddle weeping, whose gentle touch
upon their fevered brows calms and soothes them.
This is what I am warning you about: never mind

the swarming lunatics, they are everywhere, but
once you have seen that Angel in your midst
the sorrow and longing will tear at you and

trouble you all the days of your life.

(Red Hawk)

CHAPTER 2

The Mammal Instrument—Inner Processes

When you are identified with the mind you cannot be very intelligent because you become identified with an instrument, you become confined by the instrument and its limitations. And you are unlimited—you are consciousness.

Use the mind, but don't become it . . . mind is a beautiful machine. If you can use it, it will serve you; if you cannot use it and it starts using you, it is destructive, it is dangerous. It is bound to take you . . . into some suffering and misery . . . Mind cannot see; it can only go on repeating that which has been fed into it. It is like a computer; first you have to feed it . . . But you should remain the master so that you can use it; otherwise it starts directing you.

(Osho. *The Dhammapada: The Way of the Buddha*, 171)

From birth we are taught untruths, many of them unintentional, from ignorance. One such important untruth is that we have a soul. This is very bad teaching, because it suggests that the soul is separate from myself, as in: You have a car; thus, the car is a possession of mine, separate from me. So we grow up believing that the soul is somewhere in the body and is a possession of mine, but is not who I am.

Good teaching would help me to understand not that I have a soul, but that I am a soul, and I exist for a brief moment in a *human biological instrument,* a human body. We are souls having a human experience. As far as I can tell, we humans are the only creatures on the planet with two natures in one body: we are "human beings": a human, which is mammal and is the body; and a *"being"** which is not human and is not the body. Here I will use "being" and "soul" to mean the same thing. The souls who are sent to Earth are sent to a kindergarten for undeveloped souls; we are souls in embryo. We are sent here to develop ourselves, with help. We cannot do it alone. And help is always available, if I have the eyes to see it and the ears to hear it. Of all the sources of help available to the soul in its development, none is more crucial, more helpful, more revealing, or more direct and personal than self observation.

It is a beautiful system we are born into, as perfect and precise as the intelligence which made it and us. Because we are meant to function and develop efficiently, safely, and effectively in this school for souls, this kindergarten, the curriculum is designed not as a generalization, so that one-size-fits-all, the way our ordinary external education is designed. In this school, self observation reveals exactly what is needed and wanted by each individual soul, when it is needed, how it is needed, and at what speed it will be implemented. We do not learn at the same pace. Very intelligent people may learn slowly. The learning which arises from self observation happens at exactly the pace with which I am able and willing to observe, no more, and no faster. Thus it is safe and it is tailored precisely to the needs of each individual soul. I am in charge of the amount and the pace at which I learn.

The first thing which needs to be understood, and this will be repeated in many different ways throughout this owner's manual because it is difficult for the human mind to believe, is this: the act of self observation is the only change a human being needs to make in her behavior; everything else, all fundamental changes in behavior, emotion, and thinking arise as a by-product of this practice. In other words, self observation is radical, revolutionary, evolutionary, and fundamental change in the inner world of the human biological instrument. Werner Heisenberg was a twentieth-century German physicist. He had an insight which altered the way we see physics, and this insight was called "Heisenberg's uncertainty principle." It said simply this: The act of observation changes the thing observed. And this proved to be true on the micro, as well as on the macro level, from the observation of subatomic particles to the observation of galaxies. The laws of physics and the laws of metaphysics are identical; physics describes external laws, metaphysics internal laws. Thus, self observation changes what is observed within. I do not have to change anything; in fact, to attempt to do so is error and leads to trouble. I don't know what to change or how to change it.

All I have to do is observe myself honestly and without judgment.

We are souls in a mammal body. The body has inner functions, among which are intellectual, emotional, instinctive, and moving functions. Each of these functions uses a special energy unique to its function and different from the energy of the other functions. Thus, the energy required for thought is not the same as the energy of emotion. This is easily observed and also this difference may be sensed as well as observed. Observation includes sensing the body, sensing its limbs, its weight and mass, as well as the energy which moves within it. Each of these energetic functions within has its own energy *center*,* sometimes called in other systems "chakras."

Intellectual center is thinking center, head-brain, left hemisphere; emotional center is emotions, and is located roughly in the region of mid-breast-solar plexus; instinctive center is located at the navel; and moving center is located at the base of the spine. These centers of energy can be sensed with directed attention. Each of these centers operates with a different energy and at a different speed. To illustrate this is simple. Suppose a man is walking through the tall grass to the river and alongside the trail a snake is poised to strike. Before he can consciously do anything, his body leaps aside. This illustrates the relative speed of centers in relation to each other. Instinctive center is so fast that it can break down, absorb, and disseminate one sip of alcohol or one pain pill, within seconds or even milliseconds of its ingestion, which when you consider it, is truly astonishing. If intellectual center had to do that, it would take days, weeks, years. Following instinctive center in speed is, as you may have deduced, moving center. Moving center responds to instinctive center's reaction to the snake very, very quickly, from survival need. For the purpose of simplifying things, some traditions join moving and instinctive centers, speaking of them as "instinctive-moving center" and speak then of "3-centered man." The Gurdjieff Work, for example, uses this simplification, and it is useful for our purposes here as well. (For more exact description of speed of centers, see Ouspensky. *In Search of the Miraculous*. 193-195, 338-340 and Ouspensky. *The Psychology of Man's Possible Evolution*. New York: Vintage Books, 1974. 76-82).

Intellectual center is much, much slower and after the fact. Once the body is safely out of danger, the mind reacts, but too slowly to save my life. That was the job of instinct-moving. And always last to know is intellectual center, always last-to-know because it is by far, far, the slowest of the four centers. Once I have an emotional charge and the body is out of danger, now the intellectual center grasps the situation and it begins to take what has happened in the past and project it into the future, as in: "Oh my God! I'm never walking down that path again." And yet—ponder this—it is to this center, the slowest of all the centers, the center which is always the last to know, which we assign the impossible burden of running the life. This is not what it was designed to do, but what it has been forced to do by our culture and our lifestyle. Our entire educational system is designed to educate only the intellectual center. Emotions and feelings, which are not the same, have no place in our education. Nor does instinct. We used to at least give a nod to the physical body, moving center, with what we called physical education. But even that much has mostly disappeared from our technological and scientific educational structure. The result is an unbalanced human. Every one of us is unbalanced, that is we have our center of gravity or response to life, in one of the three centers: instinctive-moving, or sensual person; emotional person whose primary response to life is emotional; or intellectual person, whose primary response is to think about things. In each of us, one center dominates and thus our response to stimuli differs according to our type or center of gravity. One response is no greater or more valuable than another; they are all equal and all equally unbalanced and inappropriate to the situation at hand.

So in order for intellectual center to carry out this assignment for which it was not made and cannot perform, it must slow everything down. To do this, it runs everything through its stored habits = predictable, controllable, don't have to think about it = automatic pilot = less stress from an impossible job. Whereas, if

I trust my instincts, I get a whole different set of responses, not from the past, habit, but from an immediate response to the present situation. Operating from habit, I am inefficient and inappropriate most of the time.

One of the first tasks of self observation is to try to observe these centers in action and sense the quality of energy which is appropriate to the workings of each center. There are more than three centers of course, but for purposes of self observation, it is useful to begin by trying to discern the action of these three centers and to sense the energy unique to each one.

The Star-Driller's Attention
(for Little Moose)

In a dark and narrow tunnel they kneel
one behind the other
lit only by lamps on their hats,
drilling holes for dynamite.

The front man holds the 5-foot drill
with its star-shaped, tapered point.
One hand is inches from the butt.
His beam is focused on the point.
He never looks back.

The rear man swings the 12 pound hammer
with all his might.
His beam is focused on the butt.
He never looks away.

The rhythmic noise of the blows is deafening
in that small tight place so
their ears are plugged and they never speak.
Sometimes the front man will tire
and wish to rest.

He cannot yell,
he cannot turn,
so just after the hammer strikes
he places his thumb

directly over the butt
where the hammer lands.
The rear man's beam
is focused on the butt.

He never looks away.

(Red Hawk. *The Sioux Dog Dance*, 13)

CHAPTER 3

How To Observe—
Fundamental Principles

Your work is to discover your work
And then with all your heart
To give yourself to it.
(Buddha. *Dhammapada*, 62)

The practice of self observation includes the practice of "finding yourself," locating yourself in time and space, in the body but not as the body, and then managing the body: this is known as self remembering. Self observation and self remembering go together like left and right; they are one thing. Self observation is a practice and is part of a system of practices which taken together have traditionally been called "The Work." That is, these practices are the rightful, lawful work given to the soul in order to develop itself in the Earth school. We are given the human opportunity in order to learn how to work in a way which develops and matures us as souls and is therefore useful to our Creator and to Its creation. Mature souls know how to work and they do their work. Buddha calls this "The way of perfection" (*Dhammapada*,

96). Self observation is, therefore, a lawful practice and a way of power, so it must be practiced according to its laws. Bad habits multiply and lead to trouble, whereas the careful and honest practitioner will find oneself always having a source of inner help in one's difficulties and struggles. The four fundamental principles of self observation are as follows:

1) Without judgment: This is the most difficult principle to understand. The mind is the judge, constantly judging every person, event, and thing which occurs in my life. It judges in order to file/store information. It does so by establishing two large generalized categories into which it files all people, events and things which occur in my life: like//dislike (or good//bad—etc.). Then by association (comparison and contrast) it judges every single thing in my life, constantly, in order that it might label and file everything. It also judges every one of my actions *in order to create the illusion of separation between myself and the action:* I speak cruel words, then I judge those words as wrong and in so doing, I create the illusion that I am separate from the action being judged. The moment there is blame, there is separation from what is blamed. In this way, I prevent myself from seeing and feeling my behavior and taking full responsibility for it, owning my behavior. Judgment keeps me blind to myself. And I believe in this judgment process totally, either by accepting or rejecting what it tells me. Either way, I am "identified" (= "I am that") with the process of judgment. It rules, I obey without question.

Thus, to observe without judgment means to hold the attention steadily on bodily-*sensation*,* stay steady and unmoved in the body, relax the body, and allow the process to dissolve. When the intellectual-emotional complex triggers any movement not called for by the situation at hand, let that movement of thought and/or emotion remind me to steady and stabilize the attention on bodily sensation—be present in the body without grabbing hold of ("identifying with") the thought or emotion: find myself, manage the body. Then see what happens to the energy of thought/emotion when I do not follow it or allow it to capture the attention. Like a doe hidden in tall grass when the hunter is stalking, let the attention remain absolutely motionless, steady, stable and unmoving in the midst of the intellectual-emotional-complex searching for the attention, in order to capture & consume it for its own habitual, well-established purposes: to restore and/or maintain its patterns.

The law of maintenance: What goes unfed weakens; what gets fed grows stronger. Either the intellectual-emotional-complex feeds on the attention and grows stronger, while the attention grows weaker, is caught by every easy breeze, easily distracted and taken by every stray thought//emotion; or the attention feeds on the intellectual-emotional-complex and grows stronger, more stable, able to hold steady for longer periods of time, able to avoid distraction, able to remain free and stable in the midst of the fiercest intellectual//emotional storms. The *aim** for the mature soul is a *free and stable attention* even at the moment of the body's death. The soul is attention; It does not pay attention, it *is* attention (consciousness). I am attention.

2) **Without changing what is observed**: This is also difficult to understand because the urge to change what I observe in my behavior is a trap which keeps me enslaved in an unending cycle of guilt and blame. It is the judge which tries to change what is observed—this command judgment to change behavior immediately captures the attention and throws it into a state of "identification" with what is observed. The attention is no longer free and stable, but captured and consumed by the judgmental

mind, which by association (comparison and contrast) is labeling and filing the behavior in its vast warehouse of "like//dislike" or "good//bad"—etc. The moment I am taken by the labeling of behavior as "bad" then I cease to observe. Now I am that which judges and the attention is consumed by that. I can no longer give free attention to the inner functions of the body, but attention is caught by the judgment. Since I am now identified with the behavior, and the behavior is judged "bad" then the command is to change myself, as in: "I've got to stop smoking. Smoking is bad." In itself this may be true, but with identification, the message is "I am bad and I've got to change." The judgment feeds upon attention; habit must be fed to stay alive and grow.

But, when the attention remains stable and steady, fixed upon bodily sensation and keeping the body relaxed then the judge has nowhere to go except to feed the stable and steady attention. Thought and emotion = energy in the body. The first law of matter (Newtonian physics) is: matter (which is energy) is neither created nor destroyed, only transformed. Thus, when there is an influx of energy into the body (which is constant: "Give us this day our daily bread" as the Gospels language it) this energy is captured (stolen) by the intellectual-emotional-complex and used to enact its psycho-dramas. The energy has to go somewhere, by law, so if it is not consumed by the intellectual-emotional-complex as psycho-drama, then it must be transformed into food for the attention according to law. The psycho-drama is as follows: struggle to change myself, based on the judgment "I'm no good/bad/wrong" = a lifetime of drama to change what I am. The alternative is to observe without "identification" with the judgmental process, accepting whatsoever I see, allowing it to be in the body, and not doing anything about it at all—simply observing, relaxing, accepting, allowing—neither for nor against. In the ancient spiritual schools this practice was called "*neti–neti*" = "not this–not that." In the shamanic schools, this practice was known as "not-doing." It was also called "stopping the world." It is a mature soul who understands and follows the law of attention. One who does not follow the law is a prisoner, a slave, enslaved by "identification" to a lifetime of doing exactly as one is told by the judge, without question, unwavering suffering and sorrow. This constant identification with the judgment process is known as "*contamination.*"*

3) With attention on bodily sensation and a relaxed body: No observation without sensation is another way of putting this principle. This is called in some traditions "self remembering." That is, it is the first and initial stage of self remembering: I find myself. Self observation alone is not enough, if I do not also remember myself—that is, when I observe, first I must find myself, I must locate myself in time and space, in the body, in the present. At the same time as I am observing, I keep part of my attention focused on bodily sensation. There is always sensation in the body; it can be experienced from inside the body and from outside it observing it, both ways. But unless I can ground the observation by keeping attention on bodily sensation (the sensation of energy moving in the body, the sensation of thought moving, the sensation of emotion moving, the sensation of physical tension in the musculature, the sensation of relaxation, of sleepiness, the sensations coming into the machine via the five senses: sight, smell, taste, touch, sound—all of this is what is meant by "sensation") then the observation is from intellectual center only. Therefore, it is not grounded and simply adds to the insanity. It leads to imagination such as: look at me, I am "working" now; or: look at me, I am in "the Work" and I "work" all the time. Like that.

The mind will lie. It will imagine Work is taking place when none is. Thus the first three laws of self observation:

1) Self observation without judgment.
2) Don't change what is observed.
3) No observation without sensation.

The attention must remain grounded = present, focused on what is right in front of me. What better way than to focus on the body, through which all "impressions" flow. The body is always and only in the present; the body is a present-phenomenon only. The mind wanders out of the present, the rest of the body does not. Sensation is always a present-phenomenon only. I must remember that "I am here now" in this place, in this moment. Otherwise it is merely imagination, pretending, all from the intellect and without real grounding or presence. There is always sensation in the body. Feel the limbs (try to sense the right big toe without looking at it), sense the body's weight and mass. Another good practice for sensing the body is to keep both feet on the ground and keep the spine straight and in a good, relaxed posture. This is called "the practice of bodily sensation," because it will a) immediately return the attention (which is what I am) to the body, it will ground it, it will place the attention in its ground which is the body; b) it will focus the attention upon the body and its sensations; c) it will shift the focus of the attention away from mind and mood, and place it in the present, from where I have the possibility of freedom to choose instead of the present mood choosing for me, speaking for me, and acting for me.

In other words, I may at that moment be a human being, and not a robotic, habitual machine on automatic pilot. The effort is always and in everything to free the attention (which is what I am) so that it is not captured and consumed by the body's force of habits, but is free to choose from aim, not mood. Most human beings' attitude is determined by their mood, thus they are slaves to mood. It is mood which thinks for them, speaks for them, and acts for them. Mood is like the weather—a cloud in the sky is not my concern, nor can I do anything about it but merely observe it; likewise, mood is the inner weather, a cloud which is passing through the inner sky. It is not me, it does not need to affect me in any way, and just like the cloud, it is not any of my business or concern. Thus, for the mature soul, mood does not decide attitude. I am free to choose my attitude at any moment, regardless of circumstances internal or external. Any time I am in emotional conflict of any kind, there is the practice of bodily sensation to help me not identify: turn attention to sensing the body inside and out. This is self observation with self remembering.

4) Ruthless self honesty (from Mister Lee Lozowick's teaching) also means: tell the truth about myself, no matter how bad it makes me look. This kind of honesty is crucial in self observation. Without it, we join the mass of humanity, whose main concern is looking good in front of others. So this "ruthless self honesty" can be called the fourth law of self observation because it keeps me honest and in the process produces a beautiful by-product which is humility. Humility is a gift, it is grace, and it comes to one who works on self in an honest way. It is easy for me to lie to myself and I do it all the time. I have an image of self which sees self as righteous, fine, noble, all of the admirable virtues; or it may be that the image is bad, ugly, as in "I'm no good." Both are false, because both are partial, not complete. I pretend to be this in front of others as well. And I am blind inside to my own contradictions. It is these habits of behavior which contradict this self-image which my lying prevents me from see-ing and suffering. When I practice "ruthless self honesty" I will learn what *voluntary suffering** means, because I will begin to see my contradictions without lies or judgment, simply as they are in me. And I will suffer. The Work asks me to stand in this pain, doing nothing, trying to change nothing, judging nothing, simply feeling the pain totally without judging it good or bad, right or wrong. Simply stand in the pain and allow it to be sensed throughout the body. Emotional or psychological pain is energy in the body. Nothing else. The body knows what to do with the energy but only *when I do not interfere.* But my habits interfere: I think about the pain, I react to the pain, I judge the pain, I fight the pain, I try to "fix" the pain, it goes on and on. By my habitual behavior, I interfere. Thus, the pain gets worse; it gets magnified. But if I simply stand in the pain, not doing, sensing the body and the pain, then the body transforms the energy. By identification I feed the pain; by observing without judgment and standing in the pain, sensing it in the body, it feeds me: this is a meta-physical equation. In Newtonian physics, the first law of motion states: "An object in motion [pain] tends to stay in motion, unless an outside force [self observation without judg-ment] acts upon it."

Mister E.J. Gold has said, "The human biological machine is a transformational apparatus." It knows what to do with the energy if I do not interfere. See this one time and you will never have the same relationship with your emotional pain again, cannot. Because clarity will have entered into the equation, and once clar-ity enters, even one time, I cannot be the same again. It does not mean the habits cease. Of course not. But *my relationship to the habit is different.* This makes all the difference in the world.

Honesty

If you want to see what real honesty is
look no further than the dog.
The dog doesn't give a damn for looking good

but will hunch the leg of the Queen's mother
if it feels like it. The dog
doesn't care what the hell you think, it will

lick its balls in the presence of the Pope
if that is what it has a mind to do.
The dog does not stand on position, power,

wealth or fame of any kind. He will
bite the rump of the Emperor if he
tries to pick up the dog's food; the dog

will lift its leg on the whitewall tire
of the Prime Minister's limousine or
shit on the Dalai Lama's prayer rug

because he is a dog and that
is what dogs do and
in some secret uncorrupted part of the self

we admire this honesty in dogs, because
we see it is absent in ourselves and
we know that such honesty

comes with a terrible price in this world.

(Red Hawk. *Wreckage With A Beating Heart,* 190)

CHAPTER 4

Will of Attention

Self Observation is very difficult. The more you try, the more clearly you will see this.

At present you should practice it not for results but to understand that you cannot observe yourselves.

. . .When you try, the result will not be, in the true sense, self observation. But trying will strengthen your attention.

(G.I. Gurdjieff. *Views From The Real World*, 88)

I am attention (consciousness), nothing else. The soul is only attention. As I am now, attention is very weak, damaged by all sorts of external influences. Mister Gurdjieff continued in the talk quoted above by saying, "Self observation is only possible after acquiring attention" (*Views*. 90). We are badly damaged beings in the twenty-first century. We have poisoned the earth's environment, thus we are subject to deadly environmental illnesses such as cancer, which is in epidemic proportion around the planet. What is more, our technology is out of control because it is not utilized consciously, therefore appropriately. Television and computers have badly damaged, nearly destroyed, the attention-function in human beings. Our neural development, from a very early age, is thwarted by exposure to TV and computers; the brain entrains (mimics) the rapid shifting of images on the screen and the billions of complex neural connections which occur after birth and in the first three years of life, those subtle connections which make sustained attention possible, the ability to hold the attention for long periods on a single object or process, are damaged or destroyed. Instead we get an attention programmed to rapid shifts and constant movement. We get a race of hyperactive humans with severe attention deficit disorder. We also get a race of humans with a passive intelligence, programmed not to solve problems by moving through a series of steps from point A to point D, but instead programmed to be given the answers by either clicking a mouse or being told by the announcer, instant gratification. We do not think for ourselves; we no longer know how to think.

Furthermore, because our attention-function is badly damaged, we cannot hold attention on an object or process for any length of time. Our attention constantly shifts. Our minds race. Our emotions are hooked on action, movement, and thrill. Thus, it is nearly impossible to practice self observation at first. Our attention is simply incapable of it. It is constantly diverted by thought and emotion and external stimuli. We wander in and out of consciousness, remaining mostly in an unconscious, mechanical, automatic-pilot state. Because of this condition, the Work says that humans cannot "do." It means that I cannot make a conscious choice, hold to that choice over a long period of time without deviation, and arrive at a successful conclusion. Instead, I constantly start projects, actions, or relationships and then abandon them unfinished. Even worse, I begin with one intention and end having done the opposite. See how this applies to your relationships.

I lack real *will*.* I have no will of my own. Instead I am a creature of habit: habit thinks for me, habit speaks for me, and habit acts for me, in my name. I do not choose, habit chooses for me. I have no will of my own. I am a machine, a puppet, directed by habits placed in me by others when I was a child, driven by borrowed knowledge and belief systems not of my own devising. I am an unconscious being, asleep inside and unable to act on my own. What is more, I do not see this. In fact, to suggest this to people would arouse instant anger, hostility, and denial. We do not see ourselves because we do not know how to observe ourselves. I cannot see that I lack will because to do so would require the most ruthless self honesty, and for a long time I will not be capable of such honesty. Only patient, careful, honest self observation over a long period of time will give me the will to such honesty.

However, the situation is not hopeless, only nearly so. As I am now, as we all are in our present state, I do have one kind of will, either in the body or in the feeling, and this is called in some traditions "will of attention." However damaged my attention-function is, still it is possible for me to pay at least a minimal kind of attention to my inner processes of thought, emotion, bodily sensation, and movement. I can begin to notice my moods and how they shift. I can begin to notice my postures, how I sit, how I walk, my tone of voice, and my facial expressions. I can notice negative emotions. These provide me with a beginning practice in order to *repair my attention-function*. Only through sustained and honest struggle to observe will my attention grow and develop. If it is true that "I am attention", then the development of attention is the development of the soul, and that is the task set forth for me upon taking a human body. It is why I am sent here to Earth, to develop as a soul through practical work on self.

Through will of attention, at first I can only observe with *hindsight*. That is, I will see that I was caught in a habitual thinking, emotional, or physical process and carried along in it without being conscious of it. I was identified with the habit and controlled by it. Judgment will follow. I will often be trapped by it and identified with it as well, thus carried rapidly into more unconscious habitual behavior. But there will be moments, soon after or long after, when I can observe what has happened to me: "I snapped at him again when he _____ (fill in the blank)." And I can feel inside what this habit does to me and to my relationships. Thus, observation from hindsight begins to reveal patterns of behavior which I can become more conscious of. This is called "voluntary suffering" because no one can force me to observe my past behavior with hindsight. I must choose consciously to look, to see, and to suffer my own behavior towards self and others. This is suffering of one kind, and it is different from the mechanical suffering stemming from habitual behavior, unconscious and endless. Instead, this is conscious suffering.

After a long time, attention will be strengthened and I can have brief moments of clarity *in the moment of identification*. This is different from observation in hindsight. Though I may not have the will to stop the behavior in that moment, I will see very clearly that I am once again caught in an old habit pattern which I now can begin to recognize. This is observation in the moment, and is the result of patient observation over a long period of time, so that I am coming to Know Myself. Finally, after much longer patient and honest self observation, there will be moments when I can observe with *foresight*. That is, in the moment of identification with a habitual pattern of behavior, I will recognize it by observation, will remember myself in that moment (find myself), and be able to change direction because I know where such behavior is headed, it is always the same. This is the embryonic state of real will. This is the second stage of *self remembering*; if the first stage is focusing the attention on bodily sensation, then this stage is coming to bodily sensation *while in the midst of identification with a mood, emotion, movement, or habitual behavior.* This is the further maturation of the will of attention, which occurs as the soul matures and develops through the Work practice of self observation and self remembering.

Eventually, after long practice, observation with *foresight* blooms into its full maturity: in this mature stage of self observation, the moment the energy of an incoming impression enters the body there is awareness, an alert attention, and before the intellectual-emotional-complex can grab the energy and use it for its own agendas, attention is calmly focused on bodily sensation; I remember myself. Thus there is no interference with the incoming energy of impressions and the body is able to act in its higher function as an "energy transformation instrument." It transforms the coarser energy of entering impressions into the finer energy needed to Work, to observe, and to love.

So in the beginning, though my attention is weak and my will is also, there is the seed form in me, this will of attention which I can use to help myself develop. It is by the grace of the Creator that such a thing is given to all of us. Very few learn how to use it to develop and mature.

The Development of Attention

We are caught by every vagrant breeze,
our lives a constant distraction from what is
right in front of us, our vision

always on tomorrow so that
we miss the glory of today.
But there are the few who understand

that the doorway to the Divine
lies in the cultivation of a present-Attention,
a facility for seeing what is

right in front of me.
Louis Agassiz, the Harvard naturalist,
was once asked what he had done

with his summer vacation.
I traveled far and wide,
he said. How far, he was asked?

I got
half way across
my back yard, he replied.

(Red Hawk. *Wreckage*, 154)

CHAPTER 5

What To Observe

Instead of using the mind to analyze what's arising . . . we can simply observe what is arising . . . because in that observation there is knowledge and wisdom . . . Knowledge is the depth of our being and we get to knowledge through observation—clear, honest, unbiased observation.
(Lee Lozowick. *Feast or Famine: Teachings on Mind and Emotions,* 120)

The intellectual-emotional-complex demands with urgency that I identify with it and then express its desire of the moment = whatever "i" is arising and crying for attention. It asks me to separate, invites and urges separation from the grounded consciousness which I am and in which I reside. It invites suffering. And I gladly, eagerly do its wishes.

The practice of self observation simply asks me to find myself (self remembering) and then manage the body: be still, stay in place, and notice what is arising moment to moment in the human biological instrument, without interfering in any way with what is observed. The urge is to interfere of course. One wishes to judge and to change what is observed. That is because I identify with what I see and am shocked at what I see; I am unused to seeing myself honestly, without pretense or lying, and I do not like the shock of seeing the emperor without clothes. Self observation strips me naked so that I see myself exactly as I am, not as I wish to be, not as I pretend to be in front of others, not as I imagine myself to be, but exactly as I am. It is not a pretty sight. It is often coarse, crude, even cruel. It is crazy and that scares me at first, because it is not OK, acceptable, or even legal in our society to be crazy. We have a place for people like that and I don't want to go there. So I create clever masks, disguises, subterfuges, acts, and games (at least to myself I believe they are clever, though others are rarely fooled for long by them) in order to hide my own neuroses and keep me out of jail or a mental institution. People do not wish to know themselves for the simple reason that seeing myself as I am is often too shocking, overwhelming, unbearable, heart breaking.

This is where the beauty of the self observation practice becomes clear: I cannot see too much too soon, I can only see as much as I wish to see at any given moment before my defense mechanisms, created over years and years of habit, shield me from myself. Then once again, I am asleep inside, unconscious, a creature of habit. These habits are not wrong or bad. They have served a most useful function given the society in which I am raised: they have kept me from harm (unless of course that is what I wish for, in which case they will faithfully place me in harm's way), out of jail, and out of mental institutions. They have served to protect what is fragile, soft, tender, and vulnerable within. But there comes a time when such subterfuges no longer serve. They harm relationship and cause me to live well beneath my potential, masking my abilities, sapping my strengths, and hiding my beauty—often from me alone so that I cannot see. Let's face it, in most societies beauty is as likely to come under attack as ugliness. Both are threats to the status quo.

So at some point in my life I am likely to ask the key question which unlocks the gate to the spiritual life: "Is this all there is to life?" That question can eventually lead me to a real master, a spiritual practice, and to the deep desire to know myself. I have already suggested some very basic beginning things that I may observe in myself (see chapters 3 and 4). Furthermore, there are some fundamental generalizations about what to observe in myself which are useful. What follows is a basic guideline for things to notice, without interference, as I proceed with my daily life. Noticing is enough. These things will tend to regulate themselves if I do not fight, judge, condemn, or interfere with them. They exist for a reason and that reason is that they served me, at some point in my life, as protection. No need to condemn them. Simply relax and notice them as they arise, without trying to "fix" them or "do something" about them. Remember Heisenberg's uncertainty principle: The act of observation changes what is observed. This is such a simple understanding of my situation, and the beauty of the tool I am given as my birthright: the ability to self observe. One tool does the job; a good mechanic learns to master the use of one's tools and keeps them in good working order, understanding which tool is the right tool for the job. If one is seeking development, maturation, and transformation of oneself as a soul, then self observation is the tool of choice, always has been as long as humans have been on the Earth.

Try to Observe the Following in Yourself

1) Unnecessary tension anywhere in the body: "Unnecessary tension" = more muscular tension than is required to perform the task at hand (clenching the jaw as I lift, tense face, teeth, neck, back, etc). With attention focused on the body (= "*honest body*"*) then the attention is free, it is not captured and devoured by thought and emotion. This is basic self remembering and is an essential accompaniment to self observation. I wish to remember who I am, who it is who is observing, and what is being observed. So the practice of sensing the body, placing attention on bodily sensation, is enormously useful, helpful, and crucial to the practice of self observation. It grounds the practice and removes the charge from what is observed. Otherwise the charge, either emotional or intellectual, will capture the attention (which is what I am—I am consciousness) and consume it every time. It gives me the slightest objective distance from what is being observed, and in that slight space created by placing the attention on sensation, lies my freedom from identification.

If you cannot sense the whole body all together, then begin with its parts. As you sit in the morning, begin with the right arm, shoulder to fingertips, sense the whole arm from within, the subtle movement of energy within the arm, its weight and mass, relax the arm; then move to the right leg, hip to toe tip, relax the leg, then to left leg, left arm, torso, chest, spine, and back, neck, face, skull, breathing into each part, relaxing as you go; begin again. Once the body is relaxed, then observe the following:

2) Unnecessary thinking: "Unnecessary thought" = any thinking which is not solving a technical problem or communicating with others, not related to what is happening in the moment: when I walk, there is just walking, no thought necessary; when I exercise, there is just the movement of the body, no thinking necessary; when I eat, just eat; when I stand, just stand: like that—unnecessary thought can simply become a trigger, an internal "reminding factor" to help me refocus the attention on keeping the body relaxed. In this way, thought does not catch the attention and carry it off, capture it and consume it. As I am, I am easily fascinated by thought, enamored of it, and almost totally dependent upon it to run my life. This is the result of bad education, from birth on. Thought has its place and is a most useful tool. It is a marvelously obedient servant, but a cruel, ruthless, and inefficient master. It is not meant to be the master, and yet our education system trains it to be exactly that. It is not capable of doing what we ask of it, so it "breaks down" constantly, and is both ineffective and inefficient at running my life.

3) **Inappropriate emotion**: "Inappropriate emotion" = any emotion which is more than is appropriate to the present situation, extreme, dramatic reaction, not related to the present moment (as in imagination, daydreaming), not appropriate response to the present moment. Inappropriate emotion can simply become a trigger, an internal "reminding factor" to help me refocus the attention on keeping the body relaxed, so the emotion does not catch the attention and carry it off, capturing and consuming it.

4) **Habit:** This is harder to see, but with patient non-interfering observation, over a long period of time, patterns will begin to emerge. If I travel down the same neural and emotional pathways 10,000 times or more, even an idiot such as me will begin to notice that I have been here before, and *always with the same result*! That is because habit repeats, thus it is predictable. One very clear and useful definition of insanity is this: repeating the same action and expecting different results. And yet this is what the ordinary person spends an entire lifetime doing, repeating the same intellectual, emotional, and physical habits over and over again and wishing for some different result. Seeing the patterns of my inner life, noticing how things repeat, sensing the boredom

and monotony of such a second-hand life, a longing for what is real and true begins to arise in me. This longing comes from being. The being begins to stir and awaken just a little.

What I seek as a soul is truth. Truth is not the mind's mental chatter, which is ongoing in me, nearly unceasing, neurotic and fear-based. The mind has been programmed to comment on everything, to criticize, condemn, and judge every single action, person, event, and circumstance of my life. The result is a life lived in negativity and fear. All of what has been pointed to above is fear-based. We have been raised and trained as fear-based mechanisms in a larger culture which is fear-based; we live in the Age of Terror and are made deeply paranoid by such fear, afraid of life, afraid of others, afraid of love. Awaken from this fear-based dream and I find life, which is always and only love. Fear blocks love. Fear is the shadow side of love, and like a shadow it has no qualities of its own. I cannot measure darkness or even define it except as what it is not: it is the absence of light. In the same way, fear is the absence of love. The metaphysical equation is lawful: the greater the fear, the less the love; the greater the love, the less the fear. Unconditional love, which is the soul's essential nature, is the complete absence of fear. Truth is the direct experience of life as love. This insight is gained by non-judgmental observation of what is, exactly as it is, without the mind's commentary (unnecessary thinking) or fear (inappropriate emotion) or tension (unnecessary tension) or reference to the past or future (habit), but simple, silent, relaxed equanimity, acceptance of what is, as it is. No interference. No judgment. No fight. No blame. Free attention is enlightened attention. Enlightenment means:

1) free attention (not identified with unnecessary thought or inappropriate emotion)

2) relaxed body (no unnecessary tension, regardless of circumstance or activity).

This is the state of "no-contamination" or non-identification. Here is what happened to Buddha. For years and years he attempted a tremendous range of practices, disciplines, austerities, yogas, different teachers, masters, anything you can name. One day he fell down exhausted and in hopeless despair beneath a bodhi tree; nothing had changed in him after years of deprivation and austerity.

He surrendered totally. His body totally relaxed for the first time. He was "just this—as he is" just himself, nothing else. At that moment Gautama Siddhartha became the Buddha, enlightened master of his sphere of influence (his body). His attention was not taken by anything: no thought, no emotion, just this.

These Thoughts That Are Running Through Our Heads

They always change, are not trustworthy, yet
we stake our lives on them, the heart's death-knell;
we take them as our selves and we forget
just who we are; blindly we obey though
they take us down the alleyways of hell.
Into terrible suffering we go,

until one day we see the dreadful wrong
that they do in our name. We see that these
sirens we're in love with sing our death song.
They are never what they appear to be:
they are like a woman you love to please,
until one dark day you find out that she

has slept with evil men and is their whore,
and then you do not want her anymore.

(Red Hawk. *Wreckage,* 175)

CHAPTER 6

The Left Hemisphere Is a Binary Computer—Intellectual Center

We are what we think.
All that we are arises with our thoughts.
With our thoughts we make the world.
(Buddha. *Dhammapada*, 3)

The intellectual center, the brain's left hemisphere, is always the last to know. It is the slowest of all the centers because its place in the human biological instrument does not require the survival-necessary speed of instinctive or moving center. Its function is to serve, remember, observe, solve technical problems in the present, and communicate with others. This is its place in the scheme of the body's functions. However, due to the culture we were born into, which is not a wisdom culture but a culture of power and money, a material culture, the intellect has been placed upon the highest pedestal and worshipped because it can give me money and power, the two things most valued by my society. Our entire educational system is built upon the worship of the intellect as king; we educate the intellectual center and ignore all of the body's other functions. We do not even recognize inspiration and intuition as real or of any value in the educational process. That is because they do not come from intellectual center, but are received from higher centers, from the Creator. Remember yourself weary Traveler.

In our culture the part of the neo-cortex which our educational system trains and programs is the memory function, which occupies roughly 10 percent of the neo-cortex. This is the slowest function in the neo-cortex because it requires the search and retrieval of stored data from the past. This search-and-retrieval process is linear, step-by-step, and is what we call thinking. This is different from inspiration, which gives me the whole picture all at once, which sees wholly and not in part, or as the Gospels say, "Not through a glass darkly, but face to face." Some traditions call this memory function "formatory apparatus."

It is programmed by our culture to be binary. That is, it breaks all incoming impressions into two parts: like–dislike// black–white//good–bad//me–not me, like that. So it is a warehouse to store data, or put more simply, it stores the past. And this warehouse has two large store rooms: Like and Dislike. Thus, every person, event, object, or experience I ever have is immediately split by the intellectual center into two opposing halves. It is fragmented, no longer whole. The same thing happens with the "self"—this collection of masks, games, lies, nervous ticks, neuroses, habits—which was created by the intellect in earliest childhood to protect me from the madness of the world as we know it: it divides the self into good–bad or like–dislike. What it has seen as having survival benefit it labels "good" and what does not serve or fit this category it labels "bad." It does not matter if it is destructive, harmful, cruel, or crazy; as long as it once had survival value the intellect labels it "good" and continues to enact it as habit. And the rest of the self it judges, fights against, tries to "fix" and get rid of. One part of the self judges and makes war against another part: a self-divided. There are two classic definitions of insanity: one is repeating the same behavior and expecting a different result; the other is a self divided. The intellectual center is programmed starting at birth or before, to be a binary computer, not unitary or whole. It is programmed for madness. Most go through their whole life and are never aware of the way in which thought has come to dominate their entire life. They take it as normal and natural, the constant, obsessive brain-chatter, the never ending noise in their head. We are programmed in such a way by our culture and its resultant education, that we are convinced that thought must be the master of the house.

And because of the great emphasis and value placed upon "thought" in our culture, the intellectual center is asked to perform a task for which it is biologically and functionally incapable: *run the life and be in charge of the human biological instrument.* The fact is that thought is meant to be a faithful and loyal servant, not the master. To place thought in the position of master is to place upon it a burden which 1) it cannot carry; and 2) was never meant to carry. The result is that the thinking mechanism, the intellectual center, breaks down. It is driven crazy and programmed for madness. Thus, it is "ON" constantly, it rarely stops, it chatters night and day, even when we sleep. And sooner or later, we come to see this condition not only as "normal" but as necessary to our survival.

Thought expends great energy and time in convincing us that thought is utterly necessary. The fact is that memory has only one ability and one interest: what we call thinking. That is the only thing it can do, and since it is asked to be master of the life and the body, it is terrified because it cannot carry such a burden. Thus all of its programs and functions become fear-based. *Most of what the memory stores has fear as its basic component.* Thus we live our lives in fear and this is mirrored in the culture which this mind has created: we live in the age of terror.

The mind's main terror is that there are things which it does not know how to think about. Thought equates its absence, the absence of thought, with loss of control, and to thought, loss of control = death. Thought equates thinking with survival, as it was programmed to do—it is a binary computer after all, and can only think according to its programs. It is thus terrified of losing control = not thinking. The whole aim of intellectual center is control. And it obsesses about control because it sees that my life is *out of its control* and it cannot do what it is being asked to do. Brain scientists estimate that the brain receives something on the order of 2,000,000 bits of reality-information-bits/second. The thinking mind—memory—can process about 2,000 bits/second, or roughly .01 percent of what is present in any given moment. So on what basis does it decide which .01 percent to notice and process? Simple. It recognizes and processes only that information which validates its habits and beliefs. And since it is a fear-based mechanism, naturally it recognizes and processes that information which is fearful, *even if there is no reason to fear it.*

The result is that in every situation and relationship, thought is always thinking, judging, scheming, planning, and manipulating for control. Thought cannot love. It can only think. Thinking is not love; thinking about a person I love is not the same as loving that person. Thoughts are not actions. Love is not in the domain of thought. Love comes from outside of us, is holy, comes from on High. Love is God. Thus, the intellectual center cannot control love. Thus, it fears it. It fears what it cannot know and control. It cannot know and control God, which manifests as love in this reality. The mind fears love.

So, the moment love enters the body as energy from on High, the memory divides it into two parts, fragments it. It is programmed to be binary, to work by association: comparison and contrast, as in: this is *like* these other things I have known (past) and stored, or this is *not like* things I have known (past) and stored. And since it is fear-based, it immediately, or very quickly thereafter, begins to place emphasis on what it does not like; it begins to make a list. And sooner or later, it begins to call in the past-due accounts from this list. The result? No relationship. Love dies. Love is a unity; the moment it is divided, it is no longer love.

The thinker (memory) likes to learn what it likes. It does not want to learn what it does not like. That is because the thinker, which is memory, is programmed to be binary. It is born and in its native state is unitary: that is, all of life is a unified field and that field is love. Thus, no need to categorize, name, list, sort, examine, judge, or label. But it is an electro-chemical computer and it has been programmed to be binary. It is a "like–dislike" machine. What it does not like, it will resist learning. This includes love.

Very quickly, you are going to see that much of the information which is gleaned from honest self observation, it does not like. Therefore it will resist such information, and have a hundred good reasons, excuses, justifications, and blaming for not believing it, not remembering it, and not acting upon it. Furthermore, the information gleaned from this book it is not going to want you to have, because much of it exposes the Wizard pulling the wires and running the smoke machine behind the curtain; that is, it exposes the inner workings of the intellectual center.

Thought gains its dominance and control by a simple device: *not being observed.* Please see the beauty of this understanding and how it can help you; try to intuit what this means without thinking about it. In other words, automatic pilot, mechanical behavior, repetitious habitual behavior is what thought demands. Why? Because the intellectual center does not have to think about it. It is hopelessly overloaded, being asked to be the master of the domain. It cannot stand up to the demand. Therefore, it wants everything to be predictable, controlled, and repetitious. It requires for its control that we do not pay attention to our lives. It requires us to act from old, stored, borrowed belief systems programmed into us by others, beliefs which it has never had to examine or think about at all; all of that work was done by others. To have to do this work itself would be fearful, might separate us from the herd which put those beliefs into us, and would require it going into unknown territory, which it fears.

To thought, the most terrifying thing of all is the unknown. Because if it is unknown, really unknown, thought cannot think about it. It can only think about what it knows, and what it knows is only what has already taken place = the past. Thought as we know it, not inspiration, can only operate on the past, or by projecting what it knows from the past, and imagining it taking place in the future. Thus, the electro-chemical, binary computer is a "past–future" machine. It is a "like–dislike," "past–future" machine: binary.

Remember that the computer is very selective. If we receive upwards of 2,000,000 discrete bits of information per second, the computer can handle only about 2,000 or so. Thus it must reject roughly 1,998,000 bits of reality every second. On what basis does it decide to retain those 2,000 bits which it assimilates?

Simple. It selects only those bits *which verify and validate its programmed perceptions of the world.* And those perceptions are in the form of belief systems. If it believes that the world is a cold, unfriendly, fearful place, then it accepts and assimilates only that information which proves this belief to be true. Everything else it rejects or changes—makes it up—into agreement. If it believes, for example, I am no good (which is my computer's ruling belief) or I am stupid, or ugly, or Iraq is evil, then it receives and assimilates only those bits which validate and verify this view of me or the world.

Memory is lazy; it does not want to do the impossible task to which it is assigned by ignorant education. So it takes everything for granted and is highly selective. Otherwise it would have to think about everything. This way, it can run on automatic pilot and spend most of its time doing what it loves to do most: *fantasize*. The brain's left hemisphere spends most of its time in fantasy, dreaming. And the dreams it creates, it responds to *as if they were real*. It does not differentiate between its fantasies and reality. To the memory-unit, A=A=A and there is no B. To it, its fantasies are as real as any external phenomenon. And like a programmed robot, I respond to them, act upon them, believe in them, *as if they were real*. If it is programmed to emphasize only what is good, it labels itself an optimist; if it is programmed to emphasize only what is bad, then it calls itself a realist. Optimist–pessimist=binary; between these two extremes self observation creates a third force, a balancing or "reconciling" force, a "Middle Way" as Buddha called it.

Words Are Not Actions

I have known some,
especially in the university,
who thought that if they gave a fine talk
or wrote a long article for the journals,
this made them men of action.

The Indians knew better.
Before a warrior went into battle
he would not speak.
He went into the sweat lodge with others;
they drummed and sang and prayed.
Then for 3 days he went into solitude,
preparing his heart for his death.
When he came out, ready to ride,
his woman handed him axe and bow.
No word was spoken.

Some came back dead or badly wounded.
There was a big fire; all gathered
to hear the tales of battle.
The warriors laughed and laughed,
made jokes about each other,
told true stories that were so and not so.
They knew the wounds would heal,
knew the dead would be fed to the birds.

The Indians had a saying:
words fall down on the ground
like shit from the dogs;
deeds rise up in the sky
like the spirit leaving the body.

(Red Hawk. *Sioux Dog Dance*, 37)

CHAPTER 7

The Blind Spot—The Capture and Consume Cycle

Every phenomenon arises from a field of energies: every thought, every feeling, every movement of the body is the manifestation of a specific energy, and in the lopsided human being one energy is constantly swelling up to swamp the other. This endless pitching and tossing between mind, feeling, and body produces a fluctuating series of impulses, each of which deceptively asserts itself as "me": as one desire replaces another, there can be no continuity of intention, no true wish, only the chaotic pattern of contradiction in which we all live, in which the ego has the illusion of will power and independence. Gurdjieff call this "the terror of the situation."
(Peter Brook. "The Secret Dimension," 30)

Everything eats and is eaten, this is the law. It works on every level, from galaxy to atomic particle, from God to creature, from Earth to man. Related to this law is another: what gets fed grows stronger; what doesn't get fed dies. As above, so below, and what is true in physics is true in metaphysics as well. Our psyche is lawfully constructed around a key element or neurotic fixation, called variously in different traditions, "contamination" or "the cramp" or "chief feature" or "chief fault" or "chief flaw" or "petty tyrant" or "*blind spot*"*—different traditions of Work have different names for the *ego*'s* chief or salient or central core, its foundational neurosis or belief system. But it is this flaw around which my psychology is constructed, and it rules the inner world by remaining invisible. What is more, and here is the key: *I am addicted to my flaw!* I believe in it and give my life to it. It is this which controls the intellectual-emotional-complex. It is this which captures and consumes attention. It is this which must be continuously fed. I like "petty tyrant" because that is exactly what it is and how it behaves. This was the term used often in shamanistic traditions. But for our purposes I prefer to call it "the blind spot" because this so simply and accurately describes its action upon my consciousness: it feeds upon available energy within, but is constructed in such a way as to be all but invisible to me in ordinary life. In the Gospels, Jesus says, "Easier to see a mote [a speck of dust, rh] in your neighbor's eye than a beam [a log which holds up the roof, rh] in your own." This is a law. We are constructed in such a way that we *cannot see our own flaw*, but can easily see our neighbor's. Earth is a school for flawed souls. Each of us has a flaw, which is meant to be food for the developing soul. Thus, each of us has a blind spot around which one's psychology is constructed. It is this blind spot which drives our lives and controls our relationships. Others can see it, we cannot. And a wise man knows that if another tells me what my blind spot is, I will deny it and be angry that he could think such a thing of me. Only by the most patient and honest self observation without judgment, over a long period of time, will a person gain the clarity, honesty, and strength necessary to see one's own blind spot.

The blind spot steals the energy of attention for its own food. It does not live in a single center within. It uses intellectual and emotional centers symbiotically and creates of them an interacting complex called the intellectual-emotional-complex (some traditions call this "the *labyrinth*"*). Sometimes it will manifest as a pattern of thought, sometimes as emotional pattern or habit, and often thought will trigger emotion. Thus, they form a complex. In me the blind spot is self-hatred, and it is well guarded and masked by lying, fear of rejection, panic, fear of relationship, fear of intimacy, paranoia, cheating, anger, and self destructive behavior. So for years it looked as if such habits as lying, then fear of rejection, then other habits were the blind spot. It remained concealed from me, but as I worked through layer after layer, always behind each thing was another. And at the core was self hatred. In others it may be greed, jealousy, lying, impatience, hysteria, happiness, lust, envy, gossip, guilt, blame, vanity, pride, or many other things. For me, "I'm no good" is the way my blind spot manifests in action.

The blind spot feeds and thus grows stronger. It acts in a feeding cycle, that is it has two halves which form a single, symbiotic unit; both halves always work together and one-half follows the other the way the shadow follows the body. Each half serves a very crucial function in the feeding cycle, so if self observation only catches one-half of the cycle, then this is an incomplete observation and the cycle has accomplished its aim. The cycle has only one aim: to capture and then to consume the attention. It feeds on attention (which is all that we are; we are attention = consciousness). Thus, the contamination eats me. Lawfully then, there are only two possibilities here: either the blind spot consumes the attention, feeds off of it, or the attention consumes the blind spot, feeds off of it: that is how soul develops. To paraphrase Newtonian physics' first law of matter: Energy is neither created nor destroyed, only *transferred*. I have here substituted the word "transferred" for "transformed" and it is the word "transferred" which I want to emphasize here. Throughout the universe there is a constant transfer of energy, from Sun to Earth, Earth to human, and so on. This is true within as well. And there is a lawful transfer of energy which takes place with the blind spot; it can serve as a food source, was *meant* to serve as a food source for the development of the soul, thus has real value. Thus, handled in the right way, without judgment or interference of any kind, the blind spot feeds attention, its energy is transferred to attention. Handled the other way, through identification with the blind spot and judging what is observed, the energy of attention is transferred to it. One grows, the other is weakened. This is lawful.

Here is How the Feeding Cycle Works:

I. Capture: First there is the action—any action will do, so long as it is habitual, therefore well known and recognizable; it may be jealousy or envy, or lust, or greed, or an extra piece of pie, or hatred, or arguing, or interfering, or any habitual action, mechanical, automatic-pilot. The advantage which I have over the blind spot is that such actions are totally predictable, and once I have seen them 10,000 times (or more—I am a slow learner), I can recognize them by their first appearance and know exactly where they will lead me—every time. Therefore, *I can be ready for it before it ever arises* by keeping attention focused on the body, and remaining present in a relaxed body, no matter what I am doing or what is going on around me: find myself, manage the body.

Relaxed body = honest body. The attention *can't be captured* if it is in the right place = focused on bodily sensation and relaxing the body, no matter the action which has taken place (jealousy, envy, greed, lust, sorrow, a second piece of pie, etc.).

But the ego, which is constructed around the blind spot, knows what will catch and capture the attention because it has seen what interests or fascinates it 10,000 times, it is mechanical, repetitious, habitual—it is the body of habits—and the sole function of the first half of the cycle is: *to capture the attention.*

II. Consume: The second half of the feeding cycle follows the first half automatically, habitually, thus predictably: it is *judgment of the action* (which is identification). I am jealous, envious, lustful, angry, hateful, eat too much, say negative things, gossip, etc. Following that immediately is judgment of the action = the second half of the cycle. First the action, then the reaction—this is the law (Newton's third law of motion: For every action, there is an equal and opposite reaction.) When I try to change the action I observe in myself, I have only made one-half an observation; I have not completely observed the process I am trying to change. I have only seen one-half of that process, and based on incomplete information or observation, I am making a decision which endangers me and places my Work in jeopardy, because I know too little about what is good for me, and I do not understand in what a delicate balance things are in my body. If I change one thing, everything changes and I may be left in a worse condition than when I started.

What I have not seen yet is that the thing which I wish to change, the behavior or more accurately the h*abit* which I wish to change, exists not as a separate process, but as *part of a larger and more complete cycle*—that is, it exists in a cycle of behavior in which it is only a part. A cycle is a circle. To observe only the habitual behavior is to observe only half of the circle, 180 degrees, not the full 360 degrees. The reason I wish to change the *habit* is because I have judged the habit (identified with it) which I have observed. Simple, obvious. I don't wish to change something unless I have judged it bad, wrong, nasty, like that. Here is the interesting thing: the judgment of the *habit is the habit.* The habit depends upon the judgment of it as bad, no good, in order to derive its power and strength. The judgment of the habit is the other half of the habit. The habit is not drinking, sugar, pornography, gossip—whatever I have observed—the habit *is drinking (in this case) and judging myself for drinking* = whole cycle, full circle, 360 degrees. This full cycle keeps the self in its place, in line: self-hatred in my case. This is the underlying force behind judging what I observe. The ego depends upon me not being OK, upon having problems, upon being broken and then fixing the problem, repairing the damage. The ego = problem-and-fixing-the-problem. If there were no problems, thus nothing to fix, there would be no ego. Simple.

The judgment (second half of the cycle) has only one function which is: to consume the attention. The contamination, the blind spot, *feeds on attention and consumes it.* Thus, according to law, it grows stronger: What gets fed grows stronger, this is the law.

On the other hand, attention lives and grows stronger by eating ego = feeding cycle: The first half (the action) need not capture the attention, if attention stays at home = attention *does not move from sensing and relaxing the body* no matter how attractive the image thrown up before it; the second half = the reaction (judgment) need not consume the attention if the attention remains stable, steady, focused on the body and keeping the body relaxed. It is not taken by the action or the reaction. Thus, the feeding cycle feeds attention and my inner attention (which is soul) grows stronger, able to focus for longer and longer periods of time without being caught.

Thus, the first principle of self observation is: without judgment. It does not mean judgment stops. It means that I stop identifying with it, and thus I eat it, instead of it eating me. Inner attention can only grow stronger if it is properly fed on a daily basis; thus the importance of the sitting practice—this gives me a half-hour uninterrupted, without distraction, to practice keeping the attention grounded and at home. Whenever it gets captured, and as soon as I "remember myself," = become conscious, aware that I have been caught, I "begin again." We are all beginners here. I am a beginner. Over and over during my day, I begin again. Slowly, slowly, I "remember myself" (= find the body, return attention to bodily sensation and relax the body) before I am captured and consumed by the intellectual-emotional-complex again.

Every unnecessary thought, inappropriate emotion, and unnecessary tension is acting in the service of my blind spot and will inevitably and predictably lead to that blind spot and it will devour the attention once it has captured it. Therefore: observe unnecessary thought, inappropriate emotion, and unnecessary tension in the body. Relax the body = honest body. Don't judge, condemn, or criticize, just observe. Either I eat the bear, or the bear eats me.

The sole aim of the blind spot is to feed itself, and it does so by reenactment of those patterns which feed it best = habit (intellectual, emotional, and physical). And such patterns are *always* accompanied by unnecessary tension in the body. *What would happen if,* when such a pattern appeared for any reason, my response was to immediately place attention on the body, keep it there, breathe into the navel, and keep the body relaxed? Find out for yourself, not because some so-called expert has suggested it, even if the so-called expert has diplomas and certificates on the wall and titles after his name. *Verify* for yourself or continue to be a slave to borrowed knowledge, other people's opinions and your own blind spot.

The effort to change what is observed is wasted energy—it never changes. It is habitual, mechanical, and responds to the effort to change it with redoubled efforts to capture and consume. Instead, what may be changed, slowly, slowly and patiently with accumulation of understanding via observation, *is my relationship to what is observed*—that is, I am not quite so easily identified with the dramas and images stored in the "labyrinth" therefore my relationship to them becomes 1) disinterested; 2) objective; 3) non-identified. The effort to change what is observed is the result of judgment. Period. Thus the second half of the "capture and consume" cycle has caught me by the judgment of what is observed. It is this judgment which gets me every time, and in my case, keeps my blind spot (self-hatred) intact and well fed

Judgment is inevitably accompanied by inappropriate emotion—therefore inappropriate emotion is a dead give-away that the labyrinth is casting its net. It is an instantaneous feedback mechanism. Thus, the basic rule of self observation is to observe inappropriate emotion. Also, judgment is inevitably accompanied by unnecessary thinking. Therefore unnecessary thinking is a dead give-away that the labyrinth is casting its net. It is an instantaneous feedback mechanism. Thus, the basic rule of self observation is to observe unnecessary thinking. Finally, judgment is inevitably accompanied by unnecessary tension in the body. Thus, the basic rule of self observation is to observe unnecessary tension in the body and relax it. These are instantaneous feedback mechanisms to help the soul develop, grow and mature. They are not flaws, they are gifts to help me awaken. They are soul food.

No effort towards becoming more conscious, no matter how small, is ever wasted. This is a law of the Work. Every time I observe, something conscious (attention) in me is being fed, thus it grows, homeopathically, one grain of observation at a time. Nothing conscious is ever wasted. That is the law. I am not interested in "grand." I am interested in steady, patient, careful, law-conformable efforts to "know myself." This is our hope for freedom. Hope placed in the mind is madness. Hope placed in the emotions is sorrow and suffering. Hope placed in self observation is strength and wisdom It produces more consciousness because it feeds attention. Thus, I mature.

You Know What You Are Buddy

As I am pulling into the gas station
a woman roars out from behind a pump
and cuts right in front of me.
I slam on the brakes, lay on my horn

and she stops just long enough to
lean out her window and scream at me,
You know what you are, buddy!
Yeah.   I do.

I am a sorry little loser who
doesn't know his ass from a gas pump;
I am an arrogant educated screed who
will show you everything I know for a dollar;

I am a scared tense lonely humbug
willing to sell myself to the first woman
who shows me a grain of kindness;
I am a dazed and hopeless idiot

wondering how I got here and what
I am going to do next; I am a third-rate poet,
a broken and ruined lover of God,
a spiritual derelict hooked on Dharma,

a bum for truth, a pimp
for the teachings of Masters, but
what I want to know is,
how could she tell?

(Red Hawk. *The Way of Power,* 17)

CHAPTER 8

The First Responder—
The Default Position

If we are observing clearly, what we will see (maybe not
right away but if we continue to process) is that "I" is never
angry. We will see that anger arises in a constellation that
surrounds but does not interpenetrate "I".
(Lozowick. *Feast or Famine*, 121)

You are a soul in a mammal body, oh weary Traveler. Thus, it is
crucial to understand how this body operates, its inner functions
as well as its external manifestations. Mammals learn in five ways:
observation, repetition, modeling, trial and error, and play. Self
observation utilizes all five of these learning modes. The intellectual-emotional-complex is hard-wired into the central nervous
system. And the default position, the first responder in the central
nervous system of all mammals, is the survival instinct. That is
ground zero in a mammal, and it is in us as well. Most humans live
most of their lives in survival mode: any threat of pain—*whether*
real or imagined—and the first response is survival instinct. It is
the fastest thing in us (instinctive center), it is hard-wired into the

central nervous system, it is hot, and it is powerful. Its only function is to preserve the body from harm.

The survival instinct is located at the navel (instinctive center) and it houses the two primordial, primitive, primal emotions: rage and terror. Each of these two primal emotions triggers an accompanying action. If, according to my nature, my response to the threat of pain is rage, then the accompanying action is fight. If, according to my nature, my response is terror, then the accompanying action is flight. Thus, biologists have labeled the survival instinct the "fight-flight syndrome." Instinctive center is closely aligned with moving center.

The first response is always and only selfish = survival = fear-based (Thanks to Mr. Jay Landfair for this teaching). It cannot be otherwise; survival is always and only about "me." The "survival instinct" is housed in the instinctive center. We have already established the instinctive center's primacy in the human biological instrument: I feel it is the first to know and respond always (Ouspensky says emotions are faster; we disagree). Therefore, the first response to pain or the threat of pain—whether real or imagined—is *always and only* selfish, fear-based, and survival oriented; you can predict it, and you must now observe and verify such information for yourself by patient and careful observation without judgment. Why judge it? It is hard-wired into the mammal-instrument. The mammal always reacts according to instinctive center. It is not wrong. It is the way it is meant to be.

Most human beings live their lives and conduct their relationships out of survival instinct. That is why the world is the way it is and why we treat one another the way we do. Survival instinct is "an eye for an eye and a tooth for a tooth." If you hurt me, I will hurt you back, only moreso if I can. Thus, it is war all the time, both personally and on a global level. Survival instinct is unconscious and mechanical. It has to be that way, because when someone cuts me off in traffic, I do not have time to think about it or emote about it; that comes later. I swerve to avoid harm. You hurt me and I will strike back. When the Gospels instruct me to "turn the other cheek" they are suggesting a very high-level, conscious, and mature practice unavailable to most human beings. My first response is always and only selfish.

Only the human mammal has a choice in the matter when it is hurt by the words or actions of another, and only a human mammal who is practicing self observation can hope to avail oneself of such a choice. Otherwise, I am enslaved by the "biological imperative." The instrument does what it is created to do. And when I do this over and over in relationship, and the other does it to me as well, the result is a string of failed relationships on a personal and a global scale. No relationship can survive when I am constantly reacting to every kind of hurt, no matter how small, with anger or fear—either striking back, hurting back, or turning my back on the beloved and withdrawing my love (another, passive, way of hurting back). Only the conscious being has any choice in the matter. And we are far from conscious as we are. To surrender the survival instinct to the Work practice, to "turn the other cheek," is a very high practice indeed, called in the shamanic traditions "the Warrior's Maneuver." This is a rational response to pain or the threat of pain. Instinct is not rational.

But that's not what the blind spot does. It makes rational response totally irrelevant to satisfying its need to be fed. Rational response is the *last* thing it wants or needs. To respond rationally would mean its death knell. So it has a very large vested interest in keeping my response mammal, immediate, selfish and irrational.

So the person of the Work understands that the ordinary person has only two possible reactions to pain or the threat of pain.

And I understand that the survival instinct is always the first-responder in the other as well. I further understand that this first response can only and always be selfish. It is about survival of the organism. Period. That is why it must be first. It is how we survived the age of the giant predators, who liked to eat us. We are hard-wired to have this first response to pain or the threat of pain. We have no choice.

But the person of the Work has a choice as to whether I react to the surge of the survival instinct. I have a choice whether I act according to its urgent command: Fight or flee! I can choose to find myself, manage my body, observe without reacting, without judgment, without changing anything, *and keep the body relaxed* when the adrenaline surge is sent down the central nervous system, preparing the body to fight or flee.

The conscious being breathes in the navel (instinctive center), and relaxes the body. Thus the energetic surge is transformed—into a higher and finer energy which we may call love or wisdom or simply Work-energy. I am able to use this energy not to strike back or turn my back, but to objectively understand both my inner reaction and the actions of the other. Then I am able to make a calm assessment of my best and most productive course to aid the relationship to achieve its highest potential, regardless of the cost to myself personally. This, some awakened humans have called unconditional love. Along with the "first responder" in the central nervous system, but housed in the emotional center instead of the instinctive center, is what is known as "the default position." The emotional center is many times faster than the intellectual center. Emotional center's job is to measure—it is a measuring device hard-wired into the central nervous system of the biological instrument to ensure its maximum chance at survival. Thus, it works closely with the instinctive center's survival instinct. The emotional center measures one thing only: the amount of danger in any situation or moment or person; put another way entirely, it measures one thing only: the amount of nurturing present in any situation or moment or person. The greater the nurturing, the less danger, therefore less tension in the body. Thus, the survival instinct is not triggered by the "startle response."

Emotions are simply energy in the body, whose function is to measure the environment for danger or love. Nothing more, nothing less—energy in the body. Now here is where it gets interesting: there is only one energy—and it is continually flowing into the body, otherwise the body would die. What is this "only one energy"? Love. The Creator is impartial, objective love, and this love-energy is continually flowing into all living things, otherwise they would not live.

But the human biological instrument, as a result of training, conditioning, programming, is trained to identify and turn this energy into various "moods" according to the "paradigm" (= "mental construct") which it has been taught, and which works best for it to secure what it thinks it needs for survival. These various moods, when they are successful, get me what I think is necessary for my survival. Thus they become habitual; they get "hot wired" into the emotional center as a "default mechanism" so that, under moments of extreme duress, the central nervous system, and its part which is the emotional center, will immediately default to these habitual moods. Depression is one such mood, for example. It is the favorite of many people. Why? *Because it gets the attention of others who may then be induced to rescue me and take care of me = survival.* Of course, this sort of reasoning and behavior and habit is constructed when I am very small, as a result of caregivers who do not give appropriate response or information at the time I am in need of them. There is no "fault" here, merely mammals enacting their habitual patterns of response, according to their conditioning. "The sins of the fathers are visited upon the sons for four generations" (Exodus 34:6-7). That is, habitual emotional, mental, and mood patterns run for hundreds of years down the genealogical trees of families, from one generation to the other, endlessly (which is what is meant by "four generations" = endlessly). These habitual emotional patterns become a default position in the emotional center whenever there is a threat—*whether real or imagined*—in my environment.

So in one family, the default mood may be anger, another depression, another pollyannic happiness, another drug addiction, another abuse, another emotional withdrawal—absence both physical and emotional, abandonment, like that. The list goes on. Emotion is energy in the body, measuring the amount of danger or love. Period. What I do with it depends upon two factors: 1) my received and constructed paradigm (= mental-emotional "construct")—that is, my conditioning and programming, which becomes a default position; or 2) free attention of an awake and conscious person. If I am awake and conscious, then I am able to *choose from aim*. If I am an ordinary person, driven by unconscious habit, then my "default mechanism," my habitual mood-choices, will choose for me, the habit will speak for me in my name and using my voice, the habit will act for me, and I will be left to pay the consequences of such (sometimes life-changing) choices, sometimes paying for the rest of my life for a choice made by a mechanical, unconscious, habitual entity in the human biological instrument, which acts without reason or consciousness, only by habit. Depression is one such habit. It is often but not always arbitrary, as are my actions in response to it. It is energy—what I make of and how I use that energy is subject to my inner state: either habitual, unconscious, mechanical or else conscious, from aim, intentional.

Only by patient, honest, relaxed self observation without interference with what is observed, may I begin to see, understand, and make conscious choices from aim, instead of being a mechanical, unconscious automaton driven by the first responder and the default position. Only then do my relationships have a chance of succeeding, being fulfilling, and feeding the soul.

You Don't Know What Love Is

On the way to the picnic I stop to buy
an apple pie and the big bag of corn chips,
my favorites.
We get there and drink beer, grill burgers
and have a good time.
Just to show what a good guy I am,
I leave them the rest of the apple pie
but I wrap and fold the corn chips carefully
and place them next to our cooler so
they will come home with us. They are
my favorites.

The next day I go to the kitchen for corn chips but
they are nowhere to be found; I look
everywhere and then
I go in the laundry room where she is
doing the wash and I ask her, Where
are the corn chips?
I left them there to be nice,
she says, and that is how the fight starts.
It goes on and on, but it ends the way
they always end: she is in tears and when

I try to comfort her by saying I love her, she
says, You don't love me; you don't
know what love is. And I am thinking,
not out loud of course, That's a
goddamn lie, I love
those corn chips.

(Red Hawk. *Wreckage*, 20)

CHAPTER 9

Multiple I's

. . . the lifespan of the psyche is only as long as each "mask", or "posture" is in control of the organism . . . Usually about fifteen seconds. This is not sufficient time to accomplish anything, much less the processes of the collection of higher substances, and their perfection and crystallization into a real soul.

(E.J. Gold. *The Joy of Sacrifice: Secrets of the Sufi Way,* 13-14)

One of the hardest Work ideas to understand is the claim that, as we are, we are not a unified being inside, a single "I" always and everywhere the same, but a multitude of "i's" inside, a self divided, fragmented into dozens, even hundreds, of fractious, competing, warring "i's", each with its own agenda, tone, mood, and beliefs. It is impossible to understand this right away in any way except intellectually. I believe I am one, whole, undivided and I am constructed in such a way psychologically that the truth of my inner state is impossible for me to see. Psychology has labeled such a state schizophrenia and called it mental illness. Yet it is the state of the entire humanity; everyone I have ever met, without exception, suffers from this inner state.

But we cannot admit to such a thing. To do so would place us in jeopardy. They have a place for people like that. And so to avoid being shot, or jailed, or placed in an institution, we have all developed elaborate disguises, masks, acts, games, false personalities to hide our real inner state of fragmentation. And slowly, slowly I come to believe in this pretense as my real self. I will fight to defend it against attack or exposure.

I am a mass of contradictions. I see this in others, often it is quite obvious, and I cannot understand why they do not see it themselves, even when I point the contradiction out to them. Often they may be quite insulted and defensive when I do so, and deny any such thing in their behavior. I do the same. I cannot believe that inside I am in such a shattered, fragmented state.

And the result is that I act as if myself and everyone else were whole, united, a single, stable, unchanging "I" within. Thus, if X says she will do something and the next day she does not do as she has said, I am insulted, angry and believe that X is a liar, not to be trusted. I may even end my friendship with X if the insult is great enough, or even if it is a small thing. We end relationships all the time over petty grievances. Why? Because in the first place we believe the other to be the same "I" always and in every circumstance, and secondly because I myself am governed by many small "i's", each of which has its own agenda, and one of them, full of self importance and unable to value my friendship with X, decides to end it; it thinks for me, speaks for me, and acts in my name. Having done so, the damage may be irreparable. I may pay for the rest of my life for the momentary impulsive action of a small "i" in me which the next moment or the next hour or the next day no longer is in charge but has disappeared.

And if you ask me the next day why on earth I said and did such things to X, I will tell you quite honestly, "I don't know. I don't know what I could have been thinking." Or else, I will blame X and justify my behavior towards her with the most transparent and obvious falsehoods and excuses. This is my state and it is the state of every single person I have ever met, without exception. This state of fragmentation runs my life. It is why I cannot follow a single line of action to its logical conclusion, especially if such a line of action must be carried out over a long period of time, days, months, or even years. I will begin a certain line, even one which has great importance to me such as marriage, and will begin at once to deviate from this line into a hundred diversions, many of them directly opposed to the original line, until finally I find myself doing the exact opposite of what the original line of action proposed. I end in divorce, or I whore and drink and do terrible damage to my marriage. How can I do such things? It is simple. The "i" which made its vows before God and man to never part, to be ever faithful until death meant these vows with all of its heart, so long as it had control of the human biological instrument. But once another "i" gained control, all was forgotten. Or what is worse, the "i" which now holds sway has not forgotten those vows, but it is diametrically, even violently, opposed to them and does not want to have anything to do with them. In fact it curses the position it finds itself in and cannot believe it has gotten into such an awful mess in the first place. "What was I thinking when I married her?" it will ask, having no memory at all of the state of that other "i". In its world, the only thing which matters is drinking and whoring. Never mind the consequences to self or others. Each of these "i's" wants only what it wants, when it wants it, and how it wants it. "Damn the torpedoes, full speed ahead!"

This is what is happening in me every moment of every day, for my entire life.

Not just me, every one of us. One small "i" will take control of the instrument momentarily, will *choose for me*, will *speak in my voice, will act in my name,* and my whole life and the direction that life takes may hinge on that small and seemingly insignificant moment. And "I" am not even present, "I" don't know what happened, the implications for me, the importance of the choice, none of that. I am not even present or aware. One of a multitude of "i's" in me has chosen, decided with finality and certitude, a life-changing decision.

This "i" which has chosen has an agenda. All of the "i's" have their own agenda. And their only aim is to fulfill the desire of that agenda, at whatever cost to myself, my life, my relationships. Period. End of story. And because I am not a single, unified, solidified and consistent "I" then I am at the mercy of whichever "i" happens by pure chance to be present *at the moment I am faced with choice.*

Can I even begin to see what this means for myself? Can I even begin to understand the situation which this places me in as a human being? Seeing this is what Mister Gurdjieff calls, "the terror of the situation." This is the situation of every single human being on the Earth. How can the president of the United States say one thing, directly contradict it, spout what appear to be blatantly obvious lies, and appear to believe them himself, and then do another contradictory thing? Because, he is exactly as you and I—a multitude of "i's", each with its own agenda, and he is ruled by these "i's", exactly as you and I are.

And these "i's" are of three types:

1) one type knows very well that such a thing as the Work exists, and it is vehemently, even violently opposed to the aims of the Work; it resists self observation strongly because it under-

stands in some way that to do so would expose its agendas, contradictions, and beliefs for what they are;

2) a second type does not even know of the existence of the Work, what it is, or what its aims are; it *has no memory at all of the Work or of any aims other than its own;* it is unconscious to everything but itself;

3) a third type knows of the existence of the Work, it is influenced by the Work, it agrees to practice the aims of the Work, and is willing to cooperate with those "i's" which feel likewise.

The president of the United States operates almost exclusively with "i" number 2, and all the world's leaders, those who control the destiny of nations, are doing likewise. A disciplined mind is the rarest thing on this Earth. It is one in a million. You watch the rich and famous and powerful (including all heads of state for all nations) on TV and what you see very quickly is this: these people are fools at best; worse, they are crazy; and at their worst, they are dangerously crazy and do real harm. Some of them kill millions. They destroy the Earth. They are us with the handcuffs of social control and peer pressure removed. They are corrupted by power.

This represents another meaning of "the terror of the situation." But the real true "terror of the situation" arises in me when I have observed myself honestly, without judgment or trying to change what is observed, for a very long time and I see that all wars are one war, all terrorists exist in one place only: the war is within me, the terrorists live in hiding in me—and they depend for their lives, their very existence, upon *remaining hidden from my attention*: when I begin to see them clearly, their cover is blown; *seeing* them is profound change (Heisenberg's uncertainty principle).

Nothing can remain the same in me once I have seen the fact of my "many i's" and see how that works in me.

Now *real suffering—voluntary suffering—begins in earnest within me:* "voluntary" because no human being can make me observe myself, no one. There must develop within me what the Work calls "observing-I" which wishes to see. And as it is remembered and utilized by the inner being more, it begins to strengthen and fuse with the inner being; it becomes more and more active through the *power of suffering*—pain is the great motivator. More and more "i's" join forces with this "observing-I", they begin to coalesce and crystallize around it the way particles gather around a charge. And thus, through years of practice, forgetting for hours or days to observe, resisting meditating for fifteen or thirty minutes in the morning, only now and then remembering my Work, this "observing-I" grows stronger and more active.

Slowly, slowly its aim—to see myself as I am—becomes more active, begins to have real strength and force in me. The suffering produced by the practice actually *builds and develops something in me which the Work calls conscience.** We are all born with a tiny, microscopic "mustard seed" of conscience within us. But this mustard seed remains in embryo, undeveloped in the ordinary person. I may go to my grave ruled by various "i's", even perhaps religious "i's" but such religious "i's" have no conscience, all they have is an inherited "belief system," which cannot think, but only condemn and follow rigidly unproven dogma, borrowed ideas. Such people do not understand, they are often rigid, even very violent and war-like in pursuit of these borrowed unproven misunderstood dogma inherited from their fathers. They are often very judgmental and capable of great harm. They will act in the name of an imaginary, illusory, self-created god and do unspeakable things in the name of this god. History is filled with the acts of such beings.

But from "voluntary suffering," the seed of real conscience may spring. And this is the result of very patient and slow and careful observation over many years. *Once that mustard seed is activated, once real conscience is fed and begins to develop, only then will I learn what true voluntary suffering is.* Because the "i's" which I love and identify with (= I am that) will not go away. Just so long as I choose to believe in them and identify with them, they will have power over me. The mature practitioner simply does not give these "i's" the authority, to speak for me, to choose for me, to act for me. I give my power to aim instead. I choose to live from aim, not from the agenda of small "i's". And I suffer because I see over and over and over and over *just how easily I am taken by the agenda of small "i's". I see very clearly that I refuse to stop whoring and drinking (an example, not a fact) never mind the cost to myself, my relationships, or my life: I refuse.* And because there is now in me a mustard seed of conscience—not belief systems borrowed from others, but something which is *all my own because I have paid for it*—now I suffer most intensely, now I suffer in a whole new way and on a whole new level. *And this suffering feeds conscience.* This is what the ordinary man can never understand.

Only desperate people, who have suffered "the terror of the situation" for years and years, would be driven to such lengths that they surrendered all that they had to the Creator, in return for this mustard seed, this "pearl of great price." Do you understand? Do I dare to see how every moment I am making a decision to be ruled by small, selfish, unconscious "i's" and am a slave to their wishes? Do I dare to see how my life is being stolen from me for chump-change, for drinking and whoring (which means any and all of the small "i's" agendas)?

Can I see *in myself* the true "terror of *my* situation"? Try to observe in yourself the *entire cycle of a single "i"*—not only the acting out of its agenda, but the resulting judgment about that action, and the feelings about self which resulted as well; that is, the entire "cycle-of-the-i" not just one half, which is the action, but the other half too, which is the reaction and judgment and feeling about myself. *Verify* for yourself what is true about your inner state. Try to observe yourself without judgment or changing what is observed. When I am able to be aware of an "i" in me and what it is doing, greed and the "i" which is greedy, this is a moment of real self remembering and self observation.

The effort to change what is observed is the result of identification with what is observed, believing in it, giving it power, feeling "helpless" to do otherwise because "I am that." Thus, one part of me, one small 'i' in me, judges another small 'i' and says that this 'i' must be stopped and 'i' will stop it. The result? Civil war, a self divided, and the effort to change what is observed merely serves to further empower that which is observed and which "I" am making effort to change. Result? No change, habitual repetition of act—judgment of act—effort to change act—resulting guilt and condemnation when it does not change—further repetition of act. It is a cycle. It repeats. It can be predicted, because it is habitual. All habits are "i's".

Here is a good example. Yesterday I spent about three hours working out this chapter, writing and rewriting it. I felt that I had a reasonably good first draft. Here I was at home with this borrowed laptop making a few last minute changes when, with a single key stroke, I lost the whole chapter. I tried frantically to find and retrieve it. Nothing.

I sat there in a state, stunned disbelief and despair. Certain well-known "i's" arose in me very forcefully then. One was rage. But who or what to rage against? The laptop? Quickly it morphed to my default position: self hatred, the blind spot. Then another "i" arose, one which urged me to abandon the whole book project. It went on for several minutes, until I remembered myself, found myself, and managed the body.

I made a conscious decision not to dramatize the event or speak of it right away with my wife. Instead, I shut down the laptop, went to the backyard where my wife was sitting, and joined her in a glass of wine. When she asked me how it went, I said that it had been a good day and that I was satisfied. Later that evening at a friend's house after dinner, I mentioned what had happened, got the appropriate sympathy, we laughed about it, and I let it go. The next day several "i's" with no trust, fear-based and self hating, were eager to exploit the available energy. But I was willing to hold to my aim, so I sat down and began. The result is this chapter, better than the first draft by a lot. Perhaps not great, but better. So you see how it goes with me. Sometimes I eat the bear, sometimes the bear eats me. It goes on.

Tutwalla Baba

When he died at 93
by all reports He looked 30,
face unlined, dark hair down
to the ground, radiant and beautiful.

His spiritual practice was simple:
He walked with His eyes
downcast,
rarely spoke.

When He looked people in the eye
it burned them alive and
when He spoke
it broke them.

Refusing to be a liar,
Baba stepped into the holy fire;
reticence and restraint
made him a saint.

(Red Hawk. *Way of Power*, 29)

CHAPTER 10

The Denying Force—
Resistance To Work

*Learn to endure momentary displeasures for the sake of
the Work.*
. . . Make friends with the denying force.
*. . . If we are doubtful as to which course to follow,
we should follow the line of most resistance."*
(E.J. Gold. *The Joy of Sacrifice,* 101, 102)

No inner or outer movement can take place in this world without
resistance; some traditions call this resistance "friction." I cannot
gain traction, or friction, on ice so I am unable to move. When
tires lose resistance on a road, the car slides out of control. It
is the same way inside, according to law (first law of motion in
Newtonian physics: For every action, there is an equal and opposite reaction). As the being attempts to grow and mature, to
advance, it will meet with lawful resistance within. It cannot be
otherwise. The greater the effort, the greater the inner resistance.
Many abandon spiritual work at the first sign of resistance. They
have neither understanding nor strength enough to work with

such resistance; they identify with it and do as it commands. Still others persevere but abandon their aim as resistance grows in them. Powerful resistance causes many to abandon the Work.

The very nature of mind is separation, negation, denial, resistance, refusal, NO! Perhaps you have already noticed this in your journey, weary Traveler. And yet, via identification, this is where most of us have been trained, coerced, and intimidated into living our lives, in this tiny shanty hovel alongside a great mansion. As it is programmed, the mind is life-negative. It is the urge to die, can you see this in the world, in the behavior of the human race, in those around you, in yourself weary one? Can you intuit what this means for your life? For your relationships?

In order to develop and advance, one must find between the two forces of approach and avoidance, or as the Work identifies them, between the forces of "affirming" and "denying," what is known as "reconciling" force. In other words, I cannot simply meet resistance head on with an opposing force. The result is a stand-off. No movement is possible. Between two opposing forces, I must find a way to reconcile them. A third force must arise in me. Self observation and the accompanying self remembering provide such a reconciling force in me. They allow me to stand between two opposing forces, between the "yes" and the "no" in me, without identifying with either one. I am able to move neither toward one nor away from the other. This is known in Buddhist tradition as "equanimity." That is the ability to hold two opposing positions inside equally without distress or yielding in either direction. This is the essence of the Work. I am a mass of contradictory "i's" within, many opposed to one another, each vying for control of the organism in order to accomplish its own selfish aims. Between these stands self observation without judgment. I find myself, I do not identify. I remain quite still within, moving neither this way nor that. Thus, the forces are reconciled and movement is possible.

So, don't be fooled by resistance to Work. It is as inevitable as the shadow which follows the body. It is lawful and necessary. No development may be gained without it. In fact, resistance becomes a very useful guide to signal me when I am on a right path. The ego will find any self observation reprehensible and resist it with great force. The more one uncovers the workings of various "i's" the more inner resistance there will be. They depend for their survival upon my remaining unconscious and unaware. They cannot survive forever in the light of observation being cast upon them. They live in darkness. As one advances in this Work and gains greater insight and understanding, resistance does not diminish, it grows accordingly. The greater the inner resistance, the more assuredly I am on a right path and have uncovered something which is true.

It is wise people who understand both the nature and the value of inner resistance to self observation. They will take it as a welcome indication that they are onto something of real being-value and not abandon efforts to see. There is a saying in the Work: "If I see it, I don't have to be it." (Jan Cox) Patient practice and effort to see and feel will move me through resistance without fighting or violence of any kind inside, especially without judgment. Judgment is resistance. No need to fight or blame. Simply observe with equanimity and a relaxed body. When water meets with resistance, it merely passes around, over, or under. It yields in order to continue to move. Martial arts use the same idea, to move with, not against, the force which is coming towards me and to not tense the body but stay relaxed in the face of opposition. Resistance is lawful. Use it, don't fight it.

In the same way, after a lifetime of practice in this way, one may be able to use one's own death as an ally and an advisor, rather than the fearful enemy which we are taught to view it as by the culture we live in. There is no need to struggle against it or to fight. It is a gift given by the Creator. The Creator is only love, therefore death is love. Accepting the fact of my death while I am alive shows me the right way to live: be slow to judge and quick to forgive. Everyone I have ever met without exception will die. Therefore, what is the fight? Where is the blame? No judgment: that is the way of self observation.

Equanimity

To be without judgment, which is not
the same as being without discrimination,
is equanimity, to move neither toward hot

nor away from cold, but to remain stable
as desire strains at the leash.
Perhaps you have seen the ancient symbol

for equanimity: between 2 opposing Lions, the low
setting Sun sits unmoved on the horizon,
its light illuminating equally the no

and the yes. The Indians gave it no name
but said, Regard the eating of the bear and
the bear eating you both the same.

(Red Hawk)

CHAPTER 11

Buffers

*We have special appliances in us that prevent us from see-
ing (our) contradictions. These appliances are called buffers. Buffers are special arrangements or a special growth . . .
which prevent us from seeing the truth about ourselves and
about other things. Buffers divide us into sort of thought-
proof compartments. We may have many contradictory
desires, intentions, aims, and we do not see that they are
contradictory because buffers stand between them and prevent us from looking from one compartment into another . . .
they make it impossible to see . . . people with really strong
buffers never see . . . Generally each buffer is based on some
kind of wrong assumption about oneself, one's capacities,
one's powers, inclinations, knowledge, being, consciousness
and so on. . . they are permanent; in given circumstances
one always feels and sees the same thing.*

(P.D. Ouspensky. *The Fourth Way*, 153-154)

Here is how the labyrinth, or the intellectual-emotional-complex,
works to keep me from seeing: "*buffer** system." That is, an elaborate system of distractions which captures the attention and pre-

vents me from seeing how the labyrinth captures and consumes attention. The "buffer-system" is composed of many things, but there are five general classes or types of things which may help one begin to observe buffers, mainly: 1) *blame* ("not-me"); this is a classic way in which the intellectual-emotional-complex maintains its control, especially in relationship. The moment there is blame, I have occupied the position of "being right" and I must make you wrong. End of relationship for the moment. Now there is only attack and defense, war all the time.

2) *justification* ("me-but"); this is how I make myself right no matter what my behavior is: "Yeah, I hit her. Did you see her flirting with that other guy? You're damn right I hit her!"

3) *self importance* ("only-me"); Don Juan Matus, the Yaqui Indian shaman, once taught his apprentice Carlos Castaneda, "What weakens us is feeling offended by the deeds and misdeeds of other men. Our self importance requires that we spend most of our lives offended by someone. Without self importance we are invulnerable" (Carlos Castaneda. *Tales of Power*. New York: Simon and Schuster, 1974). This is the aggressive side of the aggressor-victim relationship, dominance.

4) *self pity* ("poor-me"); the mirror-image of self importance, the passive side of the aggression of self importance, the sly way of maintaining control in relationship, the way of the victim, submission.

5) *guilt* ("bad-me"); this is one of the most powerful instruments of control and manipulation of behavior, both on the level of society and on the personal level, in relationships.

These five things hold great interest, one might even call it fascination or obsession, to the attention, which is easily diverted and distracted from observation of the labyrinth by them, instantly. It is how the labyrinth prevents me from hearing and utilizing real help; it is how the labyrinth prevents me from seeing myself as I am, thus preserving intact its mechanism for "capture and consume." It has a vested interest in me not understanding what is being laid out here, and it knows this information is not in its best interest.

But it is mechanical = habitual, unconscious. You need not be. That is our advantage over it. I can learn to observe the intellectual-emotional-complex at work because it is predictable; it acts *the same way* every time. And simply by seeing, I can become free, not changing anything except my relationship with the labyrinth. Not changing the labyrinth at all, but my relationship to it = non-identification. So all efforts to see a buffer which keeps me confused and distracted, seem very useful for my work. Such things as judgment, identification, negativity, unnecessary thinking and inappropriate emotion, are inevitably accompanied by unnecessary tension—therefore, unnecessary tension is a dead give-away that the labyrinth is casting its net. It is an instantaneous feedback mechanism. Thus the directive: observe unnecessary tension. Efforts to keep the body relaxed seem very useful and productive. Such efforts are called in Zen "effortless effort," because it is not muscular "effort" to relax, but an effort of inner observation, bodily awareness, and understanding. Furthermore, relaxation in an inner sense, also means relaxing the grip of identification with the body's functions and with the labyrinth of the intellectual-emotional-complex. This is also what is known in certain traditions, such as Zen, as "effortless effort": to become actively-passive inside.

So work to observe buffers is slow and patient work. There are many built-in devices which I have created to avoid the horror and shame of what I have become in order to survive the madness of the world around me. If I remained sane and stable in a mad world, I would be quickly dispatched as undesirable, a trouble maker. Buffers serve to maintain a certain ordinary stability as we know it in the outer world. Removal of buffers is delicate work and cannot be accomplished too quickly. To do so would be dangerous and counterproductive. As I observe more, new qualities and virtues will arise in me as by-products of self observation. Buffers will dissolve as conscience awakens and develops in me; buffers will become impossible to maintain. I can no longer ignore my contradictions. And the new virtues which arise spontaneously in me will replace the buffers which maintain my false personality.

Always in this Work, the great law is: Pay attention; go slow; be still. There is no need to rush. Work cannot be rushed. It requires great patience, and this patience will develop in me as I observe. What is needed and wanted in me will arise as it is needed; help will come from on High, from that which observes me. I simply have to trust the process as it unfolds in me. Slow is sure and safe. Buffers exist as protection for a fragile psyche. If I saw the fragmented and divided self directly, as it is, the shock and horror of it would destroy me. We cannot bear to see our own madness, and buffers safeguard me from that shock, assuring that I remain "normally insane." Most of us manage to remain functionally insane. But the suffering of this madness is too great for most of us to bear, even with the buffer system, so we self-medicate in order to bear the suffering of our mental illness. Traditionally we use money, sex, power, fame, or drugs to distract us from the pain of our condition and numb us to the reality of our inner state. It is more than any of us can bear. The law of the Work for entering the "*Corridor of Madness*"* is: The only way out is through. I must pass through my madness. Self observation and self remembering are the ways to safely traverse the Corridor.

Simply find yourself and observe your contradictions without judgment or trying to change things. Eventually, as I mature in this Work, change will arise from what is observed. Only as I mature can change occur, and it will arise as grace from the practice of self observation. I will see what to do and how to do it. I will see when struggle is necessary and what to struggle for. No need to struggle against anything; I will see what to struggle for and that will slowly take the place of what is no longer necessary.

Nothing Left

Nothing interests me anymore.
The days crawl by like
worms after a hard rain and
I can sit here on my screened porch
from dawn until dark, doing nothing
just watching the shadows move
from one tree to the other until
everything is bathed in a pale dark,
like my empty heart.
Sports used to interest me but they have
been completely corrupted by greed
and a brutal disdain for the fans.
The newspaper once held some hope for me
because of the funnies, but no more:
Calvin and his tiger were the last breath
of true madness and common idiocy
left in a waste of the simply stupid.
TV is one crushing bore after another
interspersed with deafening commercials
duller than the worst shows.
I sit here on my screened porch and
all of a sudden here she comes again.
Every day this beautiful woman with
long brown hair nearly to her gorgeous butt
comes walking. Today she has on tight shorts
and her legs are splendidly muscled, the
calves curved and bulging, the thighs
2 tapering pillars of tanned flesh so fine
I can almost feel the hairs with my lips
and then she is gone over the hill.
Where was I? Oh, yes
nothing interests me
anymore.

(Red Hawk. *The Art of Dying*, 105)

CHAPTER 12

Seeing and Feeling

Genuine self-honesty, the fruit of a dedicated practice of self-observation, is the key to breaking the cycle of mind-entrapment.

(Lee Lozowick. *Feast or Famine*, back cover)

We are so conditioned to believe that when we see a problem we must immediately "fix" it, that one of the most difficult things to do in this Work is to observe without interference, neither judging nor changing what is observed. Lay down your sword and cease fighting, oh weary Traveler. To fight is a trap. One "i" fights another, a self-divided, and the madness is perpetuated endlessly. There is no end to what must be "fixed." It goes on and on. But because the human biological instrument is created by a wise, kind, and benevolent intelligence, it comes with a single operating tool: self observation. I am a hopeless idiot and yet, even I have learned slowly how to use this tool. You can too. We are made so that anyone not permanently and organically broken and ruined, or clinically insane, can recover their sanity by slow and patient work on self. It is beautiful the way it works. It is simple and simply elegant to learn and thus to grow and mature. And the tool for learning is observation. I have to learn how to learn. Once I learn how to learn, there is "no top end" (Mister Lee Lozowick) to what I can learn, how far I can go, or what I can attain to.

There is in every single one of us, even the very worst among us, basic goodness; it is the very nature of the being. We come into this incarnation as humans with it and it resides latent and waiting to emerge from its cover, needing only the organic invitation to emerge. That invitation is a relaxed body, inside and out. Inner relaxation is absence of identification, a passively-active non-interference with what is observed. Once I have arrived at this state by letting go of the effort to "fix," then without effort my basic goodness emerges. It becomes the active principle in the human biological instrument; it is passively-active. The intellectual-emotional-complex becomes passive within then.

The result is the emergence of basic goodness which manifests as higher functions of the instrument: kindness, generosity, forgiveness, compassion and the like. The only thing which is required of me, my place in the scheme of creation, is that I see and feel my inner state as it is, without judgment or trying to change what is observed.

Seeing comes from intellectual center, and is one of its true and basic functions. In order to self remember, to find myself, place attention on bodily sensation and observe my contradictions without identification, the intellect is required. The intellect remembers and directs the attention, places it and holds it. Seeing is one of its functions and when it does this, it is in its place. It must be trained to know its place. Only then can it serve efficiently. As it is now, it is out of its place, it wastes enormous amounts of energy in unnecessary thinking. It steals the energy which is necessary for self observation in order to maintain its flow of constant chatter and judgment. All that is required of it is that it *see* without interference.

In the same way, feeling comes from the emotional center and is one of its true and basic functions. When attention is placed on seeing my own contradictions, the shock of this will cause me to suffer. This is voluntary suffering and it can be intense. I simply have to stand in it and not distract myself with money, sex, power, fame and drugs. The only way out is through. *Feeling* this suffering is one of the true functions of emotional center and allows it to learn its proper, lawful place in the bodily scheme of energy transformation. The energy of this suffering from feeling is transformed into a higher and finer energy which can be utilized by the body for self observation. Likewise it has a function to feed higher centers, or the Creator, one of our obligations as mature beings, to feed as we are fed. Mister Gurdjieff called this "the law of reciprocal maintenance;" it is a higher function of the human biological instrument, a function of a mature soul.

From *seeing*, intention arises in the intellectual center. By itself intention cannot do, but it serves to focus the intellect and awaken its organic intelligence. From *feeling, wish** arises in the emotional center. By itself wish cannot do, but it serves to focus the emotions and awaken what is called "feeling-attention." Now attention arises in two centers at once, and taken together, intention and wish become the seed form of real will and the ability to do. When these two centers are combined with bodily sensation, which comes from instinctive center, now I have three centers working harmoniously and I am capable of the beginning of real will, the ability to do: aim arises from conscience and this combination of three centers working together. I am able to establish what is needed and wanted for my own work, create an aim to direct the behavior, and follow and hold to a steady, direct line until completion of this aim. This is the function of conscience in a mature soul or being.

My task as a being in a human biological instrument is small, but it is crucial in the scheme of things: I am asked to *see and feel* the functions of the instrument to the point of sanity, which is harmonious working of all centers in consort, without interference. My task is to not interfere, not try to "fix," not judge. Simple to understand, difficult to accomplish. Much effort is needed to arrive at the "effortless effort." Rest in who you are, weary Traveler, and bring an end to the fight.

So What?

Your dog disappeared and never came back?
So what.
Your neighbor encroached on your property and
refused to correct it?
So what.
Your parents didn't love you?
So what.
You caught your mate in bed with your best friend?
So what.
Your husband died of a heart attack and
you have been told you have 3 weeks to live?
So what.
We are all born to die?
So what.
The human race is on the verge of extinction?
So what.
The atomic bombs are all in the hands of lunatics?
So what.

Everything is what it is,
exactly as it is; all meaning and all suffering
derive from judging it good or bad,
which is arbitrary, subjective, relative and
meaningless.
You completely and vehemently disagree?

So what.

(Red Hawk)

CHAPTER 13

Becoming A Hypocrite

The fool who knows he is a fool
Is that much wiser.
The fool who thinks he is wise
Is a fool indeed . . .
For a while the fool's mischief
Tastes sweet, sweet as honey.
But in the end it turns bitter.
And how bitterly he suffers!
(Buddha. *Dhammapada*, 25, 26)

A good friend of mine who is in the Work recently wrote me, ". . . I feel like a raging, raging hypocrite . . ." Of course she does. It cannot be otherwise. This is the sign that *in me, conscience** has awakened. And unless and until I shift course, the suffering of conscience will torment me and be unbearable. Many seek any diversion from "feeling" this suffering. Traditionally, these distractions take five forms: money, sex, power, fame, drugs (of all kinds, including food, relationships which are fear-based, shopping, technologies of all kinds, etc.). When I suffer from conscience, the reaction of the human biological instrument—which is a mammal instrument—is simply fight or flight. Which is why we have the directives in the practice of self observation not to change (fight) what is observed ("seeing") and to "feel" it (not to run away from it).

As I am, every time I violate conscience, I am a hypocrite. Period. And I must stand in that feeling. I must feel it without running away via distractions. I must suffer voluntarily. My friend's letter was written by one who feels the *pulsations of suffering conscience,* though she does not yet know that is what she feels or why it is so unbearable. She can run from it, but she cannot hide; there is nowhere to hide. Her conscience has awakened, and she suffers. She "sees" that she is a hypocrite. So do I. I who write to you and instruct you in this practice, suffer my hypocrisy. There is no other suffering quite like it. It is bearable, only just barely. And this pulsation of suffering from the Creator does not judge, it does not condemn, it simply suffers. It will suffer until I make it right, whatever it was I did which caused it to suffer in the first place. At some point in my development, it is impossible to ignore this suffering. I cannot rest easy until I have made it right.

The miracle of conscience is just this: all I have to do is *"see"* and *"feel."* It will do the inner Work of transformation. It is doing this in me. I am a witness to its actions upon me as a being. It is accomplishing the changes within, not me. I cannot change. But I can "see" and "feel," and by so doing, I can undergo voluntary suffering. The rest is lawful.

If conscience is God—and I do not have any evidence to the contrary, nor any reason to doubt this teaching—then when I violate conscience within me, it is the suffering of the Creator which I am allowed to feel. This is a whole other kind of grace, given to those who wish to Work and willingly, voluntarily do so. The door is opened for me to feel the consequences of my own behavior upon the Creator. Consider what this means for you as a human being.

So do not despair. Continue to "see" and "feel." Continue to observe. Follow the law, let nothing come between you and the law. The law will transform you. You can trust the law; conscience is the law. It can be trusted, always and in everything. I love her hypocrisy because I understand what it means. But from one hypocrite to another, it is easier by far for me to see your hypocrisy than to see my own.

Just today I went over to my office to do some work on my poetry. I told my wife I would be gone for maybe two hours. But when I got there, problems with the computer arose, the task was much more detailed than I had anticipated, and I wound up spending much of the day there, maybe six–seven hours. Workmen had disconnected my phone, so I couldn't call her from my office to let her know. It never occurred to me to go to another office, or downstairs to the main office to call. When I got home, she was in a state, upset, hurt and angry. But she sat down and talked to me in a pretty level voice, making a stand for wishing that her feelings be considered and that I be a man of my word, reliable and considerate. I was defensive and offended, full of justifications for my actions. Momentarily I defended and excused, my own hypocrisy, but conscience was giving its still, small pulsation of remorse. And I knew she was right. Pretty soon I apologized.

Her response was that I didn't mean it because I wasn't feeling it. This was only half-right. She was right that I did not feel like apologizing. I felt like lashing out in defense and retaliation for being exposed. This was a well-known "i" in me, an easily offended, hostile, cold, retaliatory and crude "i" with no respect for the Work or others, only wishing to be right and get even. So there was that in me. At the same time, there was an aim in me to do the right thing, no matter how I felt or what mood was in me. I was committed to the practice of doing the right thing, operating from basic goodness, even when I didn't feel it. I meant the apology, even though at that moment I didn't feel like apologizing, I felt like striking back. I meant it even if I didn't feel it. So my point is simple: *do the right thing even when you don't feel like it.* In this way I deal with my own hypocrisy. This was a moment of another kind of self remembering: in the midst of a certain mood (an inner small "i") I found myself, managed the body, and remembered my aim. My wife's willingness to talk it through triggered the wish to remember the Work and act on it. Here is a case where one person's level and honest response helped me to behave in a finer way, from basic goodness. If she hadn't done so? I don't know; don't ask.

Easier To See A Mote in Your Neighbor's Eye

A gifted spiritual Teacher asks
if I will perform a simple task
with His people in Little Rock.

I think I did a fine job, so it's a shock
when I get a stern rebuke from my Master
who tells me what I did was a disaster,
no matter how many were helped, how many renewed,

because I did it with the wrong attitude;
the operation was a success, I reported with pride,
overlooking the fact that the patient died:
I helped them to see their Attention was weak,
but was arrogant when I needed to be gentle and meek.
The right thing done for the wrong reason
is doomed like the rose which blooms out of season.

(Red Hawk. *Wreckage,* 73)

CHAPTER 14

Voluntary Suffering

The seeker should be able to recognize his faults without identifying with them. He must be able to control his animal nature by mental exertion and by examination of conscience.

(E.J. Gold. *The Joy of Sacrifice*, 118)

If you want to know what real suffering is, as opposed to the mechanical suffering created by conditioning, begin the practice of self observation without judgment. This suffering which arises from self observation without judgment is known in the Work as "voluntary suffering." Of course, it is voluntary because no one can make another observe oneself. How could it be? I must, of my own accord, by my own choice begin to observe myself without judgment. And once I do so, I will begin to suffer in a new way. And it is this suffering in me which will create a new organ within, which is known in this Work as conscience. Once one has sufficiently developed conscience in oneself, one is called "reborn," a "new human." I can never again have the same relationship with my inner world, or the outer world, as I once had. Now I am able to take upon myself, voluntarily, some of the suffering of the Creator, to relieve the Creator of some of Its burden. I am able to "pick up my own cross and carry it," as Matthew 16:24 suggests. When a human understands this Work *from one's own experience*—not from what others have said—then they will begin to understand the Gospels in a new way as well. To carry your own cross is joy, but not joy as we know it.

We are exploring here together the means by which a human may recover from the wound of the heart. No one has escaped such wounds, no one. Not even Jesus himself escaped such wounds. Do you think you have managed to do so? It is Jesus, in the Christian tradition, who demonstrates the power of voluntary suffering. This is also known as conscious suffering, because it is the direct result of a human becoming more conscious via the practice of self observation. The first level of consciousness is to become self-conscious. This is what self observation does for me; it brings me to a conscious level of humanity where I may become self conscious. Ordinary humanity is unconscious, mechanical, automatic-pilot, creatures of habit, mammalian in nature, not yet on the level of a human being.

People who awaken self consciousness in themselves have arrived at the first level of what it means to be a human being. I am no longer on the level of ordinary humanity. Now suffering of a new kind enters into my life because I *see* with ever-increasing clarity the divided self, my fragmented nature, and I *feel* what this madness is doing to me. Thus, I suffer. Suffering is the great motivator in human life. When there is pleasure, I become automatic, maintaining the status quo. But when pain enters, I am constructed in such a way that I move away from pain. Suffering motivates me to Work, to make effort, to see more in order to find my way through suffering to pleasure.

Voluntary suffering arises from the horror of *seeing* the divided self without the protection of so many buffers. I see myself as I am, not as I have always pretended to be. I see myself without lying. Honesty arises in me, and humility, as by-products of self observation. That is, all of the virtues which the great religious traditions have encouraged, begin to awaken in me from the matrix of my basic goodness.

Voluntary suffering produces in me virtue, but it is not the kind of self-righteousness which is so obvious in those who show off their virtue in the public house. From self-righteousness comes the very worst of human behavior, unimaginable horrors, war and violence of every kind. No. The self conscious being has a quiet virtue, hidden from view because it arises with humility. I see what I am. I do not pretend to be otherwise. Speaking personally, I see that I am a liar, boastful, arrogant, self important, a know-it-all, a thief, a cheat, lustful, greedy, miserly, cruel, insensitive, vain, self righteous—do I need to continue? Do you see how you and I are just the same? We are all ego-driven, and this is what the ego is made of. When I begin to see this in myself honestly, without judgment, simply the way things are in me, voluntary suffering begins and this suffering is transformative, unlike the suffering of ordinary humanity. It is this suffering which awakens basic goodness, organic intelligence, and conscience. Even if my blind spot is self hatred, which mine is, and its message is, "I'm no good," still what arises in me to my astonishment and wonder, is basic goodness; I become basically good in spite of my personally created ego hell.

To me, this is grace. Our Creator is goodness, is love, is consciousness, is attention. It pays attention in me, because It dwells in me, as the self. It is attention and It is what gives attention within. And by Its grace, humility arises. Thank God! Humility is a balm to suffering. It is the embryo of real conscience. Humility is true beauty. It arises when I have paid for it, not before. It arises as a natural outpouring of basic goodness and as a result of patient, non-judgmental, honest, sincere self observation. Can you see the miracle of this? Perhaps you can see the beauty of it. Amazing grace saves a wretch like me. But this "saved" is not the result of a one-time experience in which I make some claim to being some kind of so-and-so and then forever after, no matter my behavior, I am in a state of grace. It is not that of which we speak here. I pay with voluntary suffering, and am rewarded with grace. It is moment to moment.

Nothing needs to be "fixed" here. It is only given to us to be a witness to the Work of our Creator. Once I assume my rightful place in relation to my Creator—as a witness—then the Creator does the rest. My task is to observe without judgment, "not doing," and leave the rest to my Creator. The Creator is kind and good. But, It will not interfere, ever, for any reason. It will not force Itself, will not insist or be aggressive in any way. Those who wish to thrust their religion on others aggressively are unconscious, as I am. It makes no sense to judge them or me, but to suffer them as I do myself, quietly and patiently, without show or complaint. The wise person leads by example, how one treats oneself and others, not by words alone. In the self-conscious person, a most unusual thing appears in this world: one whose words and actions match. Voluntary suffering is called in the Christian tradition, the "Way of the Cross."

Humbled By Love

You say you had a father once
and though you wished he were a prince
he turned out to be a shameful dunce,
a hopeless idiot bereft of common sense

whose behavior would shame a wild boar?
Well I am one like that, a man whose fear
wounded my daughters. Men like me adore
our children, though we tremble at our

ignorance, are foolish and without grace
in our devotion. But slowly what is gross
in us gives way to the child's fearless embrace
the way a barren plain yields to lush grass.

Though in his arrogance the proud man stumbles,
worship of his child ennobles as it humbles.

(Red Hawk. *The Art of Dying*, 50)

CHAPTER 15

The Awakening of Intelligence— Thinking Outside the Box

To be out of balance is my greatest help if I only realize it and see that "I" cannot balance myself. This egoistic wish to which I cling is just the continuation of what keeps me out of balance. It needs to be understood in a new way. "I" cannot make it myself, and as long as I stick to the wish to be balanced, the imbalance goes on. Again, only when I am overwhelmed, when I cannot face the situation, can some-thing entirely new appear that helps me to understand what is really needed.

(Michel de Salzmann. *Material for Thought* 14, 12-13)

The awakening of intelligence occurs in a human being when I at long last come to realize that by myself I cannot change, it is im-possible. I am trapped in a loop, a recurring cycle, a box. Help is needed and thinking my way out of the box is impossible. It is not possible to think outside the box. If I am thinking, I am always and only in the box. The mind itself is the box. The mind is a binary computer. That means it can only think in one way: by association, comparison–contrast, this–and not this, black–white, good–evil, like–dislike. It always and only thinks by comparison, by association; it is a computer, thus its only function is to store information from the past, from what is already known. What I call "thinking" is merely the mind's memory function examining its contents, which is the past stored as memory. And the only aim of memory is to repeat its contents and maintain its patterns. It only has one function: to think. It cannot do anything else. So naturally it seeks to convince me that thinking is the most important thing I can do and that if I don't think about everything all the time, I will die. Once it convinces me of the centrality of thought, now I am identified and it is in control. Our whole society and the education system which mirrors it is created around the centrality of the mind.

I cannot think my way out of the box. When I think about God, or infinity, anything, these are concepts and they are inside the box: God exists inside the box; infinity exists inside the box. In fact, every single thing you can name or think about is inside the box. See if you can internalize this intuitively without thinking about it. Everything you know is inside the box. If you know it and can name it, it is inside the box. What is outside the box is the category of things unknown, which is reality. This includes love which cannot be known, spoken about, or understood. We name it for convenience but it is not that which we have named. We name God for convenience but it is not that which we have named. The great master Jesus said, "God is love" but he knew very well that both of these terms were absurd and meaningless, only words, not the thing itself. However he was required to speak to idiots, little unconscious children like me, so he used simple, clear language to instruct us, which is what the Work teaches us to do. Break it down into simple terms so that our little infantile pea-brains can comprehend what it is we are meant to be doing here.

So in order to move outside the box, I must begin to comprehend the universe in a new way, not through the intellectual center's activity. The intellectual center must become passive, alert, receptive; it must remain in the mode of "I don't know," organically ignorant. This is the awakening of intelligence. It sounds contradictory, paradoxical: in order for real intelligence to awaken in me, the intellect must become ignorant. See if you can intuitively understand what this might mean. Faithful self observation over a long period of time will bring me to the state of "I don't know." Only then can real intelligence operate. Before then, all that I know, all that is stored in memory as knowledge, blocks the operation of intelligence. Real intelligence comes from outside the body, from higher centers, and it comes in the form of intuition and inspiration, higher intellectual and higher emotional functions.

When the mind is quiet and receptive—it cannot be receptive as long as it believes it knows and chatters all the time—then the mode of *apprehension* of reality outside the box is *direct experience*; the mode of *comprehension* outside the box is intuition, and the mode of *expression* outside the box is inspiration. These are the modes of real intelligence. The right hemisphere is merely the receiver which, when tuned to higher frequencies, receives the input from higher centers. Quiet mind and peaceful heart together, acting as one in harmony, receive wisdom. To do so, what is required of me is "not doing." That is, there must be a surrender of random, mechanical thought in the intellectual center and identification with emotions from the emotional center. Meditation is the most ancient, scientific, and reliable method of doing this. Self observation without judgment or interference is simply meditation in action. Thus, I make the crucial distinction between thinking, which is always and only inside the box, and the direct comprehension of reality, which is outside the box.

Real intelligence is the awakening of the clear channel between heart/mind and higher centers so that I can receive wisdom. It does not come from me, but is received by me. Wisdom is available to all, but at a price: the price is the surrender of all that I think I know and the leap into the abyss, into the unknown. This is not logical. Logic has taken me this far and it can go no further. Logic will argue that only it can lead me in the right direction, towards what is logical. This is logical, but not intelligent. If logic could solve the problems of humanity, it would have done so many thousands of years ago.

I have given two very useful definitions of insanity in this book that, when taken together, give a clear insight into my situation: 1) repeating the same behavior over and over and expecting different results; 2) a self divided. Now I add to this picture a third definition of insanity: 3) not trusting reality. It is obvious in the clinically insane that they do not trust reality, but it is not so obvious in my own behavior until I have observed myself with great patience, honesty, and sincerity. Intelligence is knowing what can be trusted and what cannot. Only patient and steady self observation will reveal what is trustworthy in me. I trust the mind's perception of reality based on its programming, but it sees *only that which validates its programs*, a minute portion of incoming impressions, and the rest it rejects.

What drives me crazy, when I see the absurdity of the world as it is, is the effort to understand and make sense of an insane world, which means to think about it. Everything is lawful. That is all I need to understand. I don't need to understand the "why" or the "what if" of things. This thinking about it drives me crazy. Instead of thinking about it, intelligence faces reality with no preconceptions, expectations, or judgments about it, and it accepts what is, as it is. Then it responds appropriately to it as it is guided by intuition and inspiration. It does what is needed and wanted. Otherwise, it does not interfere.

Thinking can't solve the problem of my life because thinking is the problem. But it does expose the problem. The mind is active because it has been asked to do the impossible: be the master and be in control. Impossible task. Thus it sits behind the curtains of Oz and operates a smoke screen of continuous thought which creates the illusion that I am in control of my life and of reality. I can go about my life as an habitual, mechanical, unconscious, sleeping walking-around robot, a proper mammal who fits into the herd, some herd, somewhere. I can continue to do the same things in the same way and not have to think for myself.

When I use the word "think" I don't use it in the ordinary way. It is a "higher order" of thought which does not depend upon straight-line logic or reason for its understanding. The mind cannot understand. All it can do is name and store information by means of association for use when it is called upon to do so. Thus, the question: does the mind have any practical use at all? Absolutely: 1) to observe; 2) to solve technical problems in the present; 3) to communicate with others; 4) to serve attention and intelligence; 5) to align with the heart. This is its place and in its place it is an incredibly effective tool. The intellectual-emotional-complex is not meant to rule. When it is asked to rule, its rule is tyranny and violence of all kinds, on all levels. It is meant to be a faithful servant of higher centers, a receiver, as any computer. The fact that computers have taken over our world tells you something about us and about the mind which created them in its image.

I Keep A Different List

My neighbor counts his losses and his gains,
but i keep track of raindrops when it rains;
he makes note of coins and dollar bills
while i am watching ants upon their hills;
while he is in the office making money,
i go out among the bees to gather honey,
and when he comes home tired and goes online,
i am in the back yard drinking wine.
My wife and i sit in the gathering dark
and watch the lightning bugs and bright stars spark
until we disappear, are covered up with night,
while my neighbor plots his life by computer light.

(Red Hawk)

CHAPTER 16

Being-Shock

*When the intensity is such that you cannot deny the death of
the neurotic mind and the life and freedom of the Work mind,
then you are in a position in which you can make a step . . .*

*We really do not recognize the fact that we have no
choice. We are totally enslaved by the neurotic mind: every breath, every word out of our mouths, every gesture. We
couldn't be free if our lives, if our children's lives, depended
upon it. We could not. We have no options—we can't be free.
We can't make the conscious choice. We can't make a free
gesture. When we get that, the horror and disgust is so overwhelming that we will be forced to choose the Work mind.*

*We're forced to see how absolutely, completely choiceless
we are when we are dominated by our psychology, and the
shock of that is what propels us into choosing the Work mind . . .*
(Lee Lozowick. In: Young, *As It Is*, 156)

Only a great shock will penetrate to the level of the being. And
this shock must be cumulative, the result of years of honest self
observation without judgment. Look after look accumulate like
water dripping on stone. It is this homeopathic accumulation

of information which leads to the realization at last that there is more to me than this continual display of intellectual, emotional, and physical habits. More is possible than this fear-based life. Once the being learns how to learn, through simple and steady observation, it finds a source of real food in this practice which satisfies its deep hunger for truth. It longs for truth and can only be nourished and grow by being fed a steady diet of what is true. And the contrast between what is true and what I am being told by the intellectual-emotional-complex and manifesting in my daily behavior is the source of real suffering. Direct experience becomes my teacher, not the accumulation of belief systems, borrowed knowledge, and the experience of others which are stored in the memory as the self, which I believe in, and which I have given my life to without question.

The contrast between what memory, the thinker, and direct experience tell me leads me eventually to question all authority, especially the authority of the intellectual-emotional-complex. Slowly, I begin to trust the reality I observe more than the reality being fed to me by the intellectual-emotional-complex, which denies my basic goodness and creates a world of fear, all to support the illusion of security and control.

Anyone who practices self observation faithfully, without judgment or changing what is observed, with ruthless self-honesty and a relaxed body, will sooner or later come to the point of horror. It is guaranteed. It is the law. It is my experience. This is what I am calling "being-shock" and it is overwhelming. I see that I am a total, helpless slave to my psychology and that it will never change. The only thing that can ever change is my relationship to what is observed: *without identification.*

The habits, the patterns enacted over and over again since childhood, go on ruthlessly in me without regard for the effect they have on my life, my relationships, and my well being. They will never end; they will never change; they will never stop. It is not their place to stop; something else must stop in me. To see this truthfully is horror. And it is this horror which awakens the being from its unconscious paralysis, which it has been in since life over-whelmed it as a small child. As a child I was compelled to comply with a definition of reality which was in direct contradiction to my feelings, my senses, and what I intuitively understood. Failure to comply meant loss of love. Now, after years of self observation, I realize at this crucial, life-changing point that if I do not take responsibility for my life, my thoughts, my emotions, my habits, and the functions of the human biological instrument, then I will go to my death enslaved and identified with my madness. I will live a mammal's life and die a dog's death. Something has to stop. It is now clear that the intellectual-emotional-complex will not stop. The only possibility is that my identification with it cease, "cold turkey" as Mister E.J. Gold has called it.

The habits are a tape-loop which runs endlessly in the intel-lectual-emotional-complex. This loop is used by the labyrinth (= the intellectual-emotional-complex) to capture and consume attention, upon which it feeds to maintain its life and its cycle. Without my identification, the labyrinth cannot maintain its continuous tape-loop. It cannot enact its programs. Memory, the thinker, the left hemisphere of the brain, is an electrochemical computer complex programmed to repeat its patterns. Simple. Its whole existence is built around this single aim: to maintain, pre-serve, and repeat its patterns. The only thing which can change in this cycle is my relationship to it = *non-identification* with its pat-terns and with my blind spot = self-hatred. *Identification can stop.* This is a conscious being-choice. The only "progress" is seeing and feeling the pattern as it takes place = self observation without judgment or identification. When I have seen it enough, I begin to understand that it is not ever going to change, it will go to the grave repeating its programs and consuming attention. When I understand this not just intellectually but also in the emotional center, when I not only *see* it, but *feel* it deeply—the horror and the shock of the horror—then there can happen what is called "being-shock" in which the inner sleeping, unconscious being steps forward to take its rightful place in the human biological instrument and assumes responsibility for its learning and its life. As long as the being is not conscious of itself, it cannot see what is consuming it. If I see it, I don't have to be it. But first I have to see it 10,000 times or more before I understand that I am not the patterns I am observing: this is the awakening of intelligence.

Being-shock is not simple change, it is a move to another level of existence, another reality; it is a change in being in which the Work becomes the active principle and the psychology and the functions of the body, most importantly including the intellectual-emotional-complex, become passive, waiting to serve. When the Work is the active principle, basic goodness emerges. Virtues arise. The being assumes responsibility for taming and training the mammal, a function which before this has been performed by the master, the teacher. Being-shock only happens when both intelligence and conscience have been awakened in the being. When intelligence has been awakened, I see clearly what is needed and wanted and I understand the implications of what I am seeing. I make intelligent choices. When conscience is awakened, I can feel the shock of horror deeply because I have become sensitized by conscience into feeling suffering. I am no longer numb. When the suffering of conscience reaches critical mass then the shock of horror has the effect of awakening the being. This is transformative. I become consistent and reliable when this happens, because

I am no longer driven by habit but by attention to what is needed and wanted in the present moment. I begin to behave appropriately, no longer manifesting inappropriate emotions. Now, mastery of mood and of the body's functions is possible because the intellectual-emotional-complex has been transformed from master to willing servant. Unnecessary thinking no longer dominates the head-brain. This is called "stopping the world" in the ancient shamanic traditions.

The beauty of this transformative being-shock is that the being which emerges from its hiding is simple, not complicated. It is not cunning or devious. It is not divided, it is a single entity. It trusts reality because it is real. It does not endlessly repeat the same worn and tired, non-functional, unworkable patterns or habits. It is a presence and it operates in the present efficiently. It is a human being. It is sane.

The Simple Life, No Call-Waiting

No cell phone, no caller id, no call-waiting, no
cable, no Tivo, no computer, no Ipod, no
blueberry, no notepad, no laptop, no
riding mower, no leaf blower, no weed eater,
no digital clock, no air conditioner, no new car;
I live in another country, a different century.

I ride my 3-speed bike to work, because
it helps the Earth and eases the body more gracefully
into its dying; it makes the body work hard and
it likes to work, likes to do sweat-labor despite
the avalanche of labor-saving technology whose function
is to drain us of our life force.

I write by hand in a notebook because
I like to see where I've been, follow my tracks back
through the snow to where I started, see how things
work out on the page, where I went wrong,
how to begin again, nothing deleted.
I don't want to know who's calling or

who has called. I've lived 65 years and I have
never gotten a phone call that made a difference.
If you reach me, that's fine but if you don't
nothing is lost.
Most people are slaves.
That's the way they like it.

After all the years of heartbreak and disappointment,
of treachery and betrayal, are you so far gone
that you believe the next phone call will be the one
that saves you? When Death comes for you,
you can't say, Would you mind holding?
I've got a life on the other line.

(Red Hawk)

CHAPTER 17

The Shift In Context—Not-Doing

The intention of the Work is to produce freedom in us. There's only one way that freedom can be produced in us and that is to choose Work mind over neurotic mind. It has to be a conscious choice, and the only way that we'll ever make a choice that's conscious, fully conscious, is to see neurotic mind in its totality, in its death. To see it for what it is—empty of all substance, empty of all possibility, empty of all creativity, empty of all genuine, human feeling, empty of heart, empty of mind, empty of everything except its own mechanical survival impetus. That's it. Until we see it that way, until we see our lives, our love for our parents, our drive for sexual fulfillment, our taste for fine food, our love of good music—until we see all of it as nothing, absolutely nothing but totally mechanical, dead slavery to neurotic mind—we'll never choose the Work.

(Lee Lozowick. In: Young, 157)

. . . The mind of the child . . . made certain decisions about his or her world or about reality based on a child's intelligence, a child's understanding, a child's expectations and projections. That mind grows up to be, as we all know, absolutely

consuming. That mind possesses us. We identify with it as if that mind were us. Sooner or later in this Work we've got to break with that mind, cleanly and finally . . . —all its elements, all its identifications, its hopes, its dreams, its wishes, and its morality . . . every single element of that mind has to be severed. We have to literally stop functioning out of the context of that mind. (155)

The dominance of the intellectual-emotional-complex depends upon continuity of thought. Break that continuity and its dominance ceases because judgment ceases. What is produced when this continuity is broken is a "shift in context." I no longer operate from an agreed-upon definition of reality, but from reality itself. I operate from what is, exactly as it is, not from meaning supplied by the intellectual-emotional-complex. This entails an acceptance of reality without desire to change anything. It entails non-interference with what is. I take my cues from direct experience of reality in the moment, not from memory which is the past, or the past projected forward, as what it calls the future. I live in the unknown, in organic ignorance, which is intelligent because it is in direct contact with the source of wisdom, without the interference of memory.

Memory is useful for remembering, solving technical problems, and communicating with others. Thus, it is not abandoned. It simply finds its lawful place. It ceases to be the master and becomes what it was designed to be: a faithful servant directed by a force other than its own contents. That force is being. Being emerges as the active principle only when it ceases its identification with the intellectual-emotional-complex. At that point, when the memory thinks, there is not inner movement towards or away from the thought; this movement towards or away from thought is identification. Instead there is steady equilibrium, stillness, absence of movement when the thought arises. In the shamanic tradition this cessation of movement towards or away from thought is called "not doing."

The cessation of movement sends a direct signal to the Creator. It is called in ancient traditions "The Invitation." What enters only upon invitation is a flow of information from higher centers which are the source of wisdom. Some say these centers exist outside of, but directly connected to, the human biological instrument, but I am unsure of this. What does seem clear is that the direct link to these centers is conscience. Conscience is the emotional center transformed into feeling center. Conscience receives direct information from these centers in the form of intuition and inspiration. Intuition is a fundamentally different form of thinking from higher intellectual center; it sees everything at once, the whole of a situation, its past, present, and future. Thus it is able to inform in a way which includes the unknown, whereas memory can always and only act from the known. It cannot know what has not already happened, thus it always operates from the past and is the past. That is the limitation of thought.

Intuition operates on a different scale and from a different context. So does inspiration. Inspiration is a fundamentally different form of feeling; in fact it is feeling and not emotion. The distinction is important to understand—see if you can intuit the difference without thinking about it. Emotions are limited because their function is limited to measuring danger in the environment. They consist of anger, sadness, happiness, and fear, and they are housed in the emotional center. Anger and fear are not the same as rage and terror, which are housed in the instinctive center and make up what is called the survival-instinct. Anger and fear are the shadows of these two primal emotions.

When the emotional center is transformed, it becomes feeling center and is the seat of conscience. Then it is a conduit for higher emotional center. Inspiration is from higher emotional center, or as I prefer to call it, higher feeling center. That makes the distinction clearer. Unlike thought from memory which operates linearly and step by step, inspiration gives me the whole picture in its entirety all at once, not separated and divided into pieces and steps. It operates as an entire circle, not a straight line.

Unlike memory, which can only operate or "think" from the known, intuition and inspiration operate in, and are functions of, the unknown. Thus they are capable of supplying information totally inaccessible to thought, impossible for thought to access. It is a common story throughout human history that great inventions, insights, and discoveries happened "in a flash of inspiration." At such moments, women and men were able to see the whole picture clearly. And it usually comes in the form of an image or picture. Thus Crick saw two snakes intertwined and intuited the double-helix of DNA. Einstein saw himself traveling on a rocket ship at the speed of, alongside of, light and he intuited the General Theory of Relativity.

Now here is the beauty of the intellectual-emotional-complex, which is not the enemy or at fault but is merely performing the functions it was programmed to perform, the way any computer does. Once there is a shift in context within, the function of this complex is to translate what is received from intuition and inspiration into language and images which can then be shared with others: communication. The writers of the Gospels, the *Dhammapada*, The Bhagavad Gita, and the *Tao Te Ching* were communicating received wisdom from intuition and inspiration and translating it into a language which could be understood and shared by others. But it is clear that these writers understood the limitations of language in this regard. Lao Tsu warns us immediately, in the opening lines of the *Tao*:

> The Tao that can be told is not the eternal Tao.
> The name that can be named is not the eternal name.
> The nameless is the beginning of heaven and earth.
>   (*Tao Te Ching.* Sutra 1)

Lao Tsu is describing the shift in context, and at the same time is warning against being seduced by words. Each is pointing to the primacy of direct experience over knowledge gained by words. Thus, although their wise counsel is useful and precious, it does not absolve me in any way from finding the truth for myself. I must verify what I am told by my direct experience. The simplest and most direct experience comes from self observation. This practice will lead me, lawfully, to the shift in context because it will gradually and patiently reveal to me the contamination programmed into the intellectual-emotional-complex. All contamination is, is simply unnecessary thought and inappropriate emotion accompanied by tension in the body, following habitual patterns down the same well-worn neural (brain) and nerve (central nervous system) pathways and always arriving at the same useless and unworkable solutions = insanity. Why react to that? What's the point? Simply recognize, understand, allow, and return to the task at hand with attention refocused on the body.

When I have reached the point of exhaustion, breakdown, and hopeless despair, only then will I consider a shift in the context from which I view my life and the world. This shift leads directly to a piercing of one's contamination. Finally, my attention must return to its home: in and on the body. Then the attention has found its true place and proper function. Then the practice of not-doing arises.

We are all operating damaged instruments, damaged by our childhoods, our life experiences, and the way our primary caregivers programmed the intellectual-emotional-complex. I am trained to view the world only through those programs, so my context for viewing the world is their contents. This is an extremely limited and fear-based world view. What is required for me to live a fuller, more complete, and more satisfying life is that the context from which I view myself and this life shifts.

This shift can only occur through understanding and knowing myself in a more conscious way: not habit-driven, mechanical, on automatic pilot, but with compassion and objectivity. Objectivity means that I see myself honestly, I know and understand myself clearly, and I am willing to take full and mature responsibility for what I see and feel. Self observation provides the vital information with which I can do this. In its absence any changes I try to make are just shooting in the dark, confusing the part with the whole, and are doomed to fail. If I see it and feel it, I don't have to be it. If I'm not willing to see it, I don't have any choice.

Self observation with compassion simply means that I stop judging myself and just see and feel whatever arises. Judgment is a trap I fall for every time and is not productive, useful, or compassionate. It is harsh, rigid, and keeps me trapped in an unending cycle of action and reaction. Unless a third force enters into that action-reaction cycle, no substantive change is ever possible. That third force is self observation and its very existence is substantive change. Everything else accrues to it like metal filings to a magnet. Self observation attracts help; it is a fundamental attractive force in the universe. It allows me to operate more efficiently and more objectively in the field of the intellectual-emotional-complex. It is the savior. It is consciousness coming to know itself, learning how to learn and create, while doing the least amount of harm. It is objective love in the process of becoming.

Often the Greatest Help Is Not-Doing

After blowing several obvious chances
to help my Guru, once by His direct request,
finally my prayer was to be of some use to Him,
no matter how small or seemingly insignificant.
Like nearly everything my mind imagines, nothing
unfolds in the way i had it figured.
Because i loved her sweet voice and
the way she bled out the tunes which
Mister Lee wrote for her, i was inspired
to write some torch songs, some blues
for her, which i did.
None of them amounted to much, but
i took them to Mister Lee and told Him
what i was up to. He said,
Writing the songs is one of the few things
which gives me real pleasure.
That is all He said. He
did not ask me not to do it, did not say
that to do so would rob Him
of one of His few pleasures;
no plea, no justification, no excuse, but
in that moment i saw my opportunity,
the thing i had prayed for.
Without regret or self pity,

i never wrote another song.

(Red Hawk)

CHAPTER 18

The Deer in the Tall Grass

To separate from the associative level, we have to contact finer energies. The higher part of the head is full of fine energy—there, there is silence—no words there—no struggle.

Where the feeling of myself connects with the finer energies, they become concentrated. This energy must never be used for anything other than my inner world. The outer world does not need it.

Little by little, and it is a long process, I keep some of these finer energies. I collect them and try not to pour them out. Then they may crystallize and they cannot become mixed with coarse energies. It is slow, patience is needed, and it is the only way to a change in the centre of gravity.

(Henriette Lannes. *Inside A Question*, 201)

Thus, I am brought slowly and quite naturally, gently and patiently, to the practice of radical presence: what this means simply is that my struggle and practice is to be present in the body, moment to moment, and to return to the presence within the body the moment I remember, every time during the day and night (sometimes even when sleeping, though not often, but sometimes—and sometimes it will awaken me from night-sleep, like last night at 4:00 A.M. with information incoming which I had to get up and write down lest it be lost). This is inspiration. It is higher intellectual center communication with the human biological instrument. It comes fast and clear. I believe you know this experience of easeful self remembering and returning home as well.

In order to facilitate this practice, may I suggest the following: whenever you are reading this or any book, but especially wisdom literature: keep your spine straight and both feet on the floor (as you are reading this) which will facilitate a certain level and kind of self observation and self remembering. To be radically present to the presence within, the essential being, requires that the attention be focused on bodily sensation (instinctive center) where the attention is anchored and grounded, present to the presence within is what I am calling "the practice of radical presence." I prefer attention centered in the forehead or at the top of the head, other schools place it variously at the navel, the solar plexus, or the heart center. This depends upon the aims of the school and the teaching. Lord Sri Krishna instructs his devotee Arjuna in this way:

> He who leaves the body with mind unmoved and filled with devotion, by the power of his meditation gathering
> between his eyebrows his whole vital energy, attains the Supreme. (Bhagavad Gita, 79)

But with the possible exception of the navel (where the instinctive center is located) all of these centers are contaminated in me. The center in the middle of the forehead and the one at the crown, or crown chakra, are clear and objective in me and allow me to function efficiently and clearly and to catch the energy impressions (that is the continuous influx of vital energy from on High, which enters the human biological instrument at the crown chakra and is then circulated throughout the instrument, or captured and consumed by various contaminated centers for their own obsessions) the moment these energy-impressions enter into the instrument, where there is objective evaluation and where the guardian-attention is stationed and remains totally still, taking in the whole of the instrument without moving towards or away from the energy which has entered: it is choicelessly aware and *not identified*. Once they are cleansed of contamination, the other centers may also give objective seeing. The result is a very efficient utilization of the inflow of energy which is continuous. There is not the feeding of the contaminants via identification (= I am that) and thus the contamination is contained, utilized creatively, not judged or condemned or fought against, not fed in order to play out psycho-emotional drama, and the contamination itself becomes a very useful "inner reminding factor" to hold to one's aims: clean, clear, practice, observe, relax the instrument. A non-judgmental, "safe" space is created within, in which the contamination may be housed and dwell, without spreading throughout the instrument. When it is not judged but given space within, the contamination slowly becomes purified.

A relaxed instrument is an uncontaminated body. Every contamination, no matter its kind or content, produces tension in the body and at whatever point this tension exists, the inflow of energy impressions is stopped *at that very point*, where it is captured and consumed by the intellectual-emotional-complex. The result is that the flow of energy in the instrument is severely compromised, the contamination is being fed its own kind and type of food, and the being is starved of its real food. The being starves and the contamination grows stronger.

However, in the practice of radical presence, it is the contamination which becomes the food for the being, via self observation without judgment or trying to change what is observed. Just as a chick inside the eggshell feeds upon the yolk—its only source of nourishment—the being feeds upon the ego, it is contamination which is ego, and slowly, slowly the ego/contamination is consumed. What is left then is being unobstructed by ego and uncontaminated by habit.

What is required for this lawful process to occur is that the attention remain unmoved (= non-identified) as the energy impressions pour in through the crown chakra (at the top of the head). Any inner movement at this point is identification. Then attention is captured and consumed. Thus, the attention at this point may be compared to a deer in the tall grass when the hunter is present. The deer remains absolutely still and hidden in the tall grass, moving neither this way nor that, while the hunter searches for his prey. Because the deer does not reveal its position by movement, the hunter moves on looking for another opportunity. Like the deer in the tall grass, when the labyrinth casts its net through thought, emotion, or physical posture, when the attention does not move to interfere, no movement towards or away, holding its focus in place on sensation, the labyrinth is unable to capture and use attention for the realization of its agenda; the various small "i's" arise and subside without action or reaction. The attention does not identify with them and they are left powerless, because they have no energy of their own. They must capture the energy of attention in order to act. But when the deer does not reveal its position, the hunter moves on.

A non-identified attention is what is called in some schools "free attention" and it is this "free attention" which is one of my innermost aims. A "free attention" is free of contamination. It is free of identification. It is free to choose, free to remain still. And Psalm 46:10 has instructed: "Be still and know that I Am God." Be still and know, or die like a dog. The choice is mine. If I breathe into the navel and relax the body without interfering with incoming energy impressions, the body is allowed to assume its higher function as an energy-transformation apparatus (as Mister E.J. Gold has called it); it transforms the energy of the incoming energy-impressions into a finer quality of energy. Thus, the energy feeds the Creator instead of the ego.

Let's say the other hurts my feelings and triggers in me the survival instinct: fight or flight. What this simple (but not easy) practice does is this: instead of trying to change the habit—which is the result of judgment, otherwise why the desire to change it?—I merely begin to give it space within, so that the survival instinct (fight or flight) has the space for its natural, biological, genetically programmed response. I give it space when the other hurts me for any reason. And in so doing, now there is no war against—so no unnecessary tension in the body. Now the struggle is for something. What? For objective attention and calm, reasonable, kindness in my response to the one who has hurt me (out of her own fear of love, which is at least equal to my own fear of love). Thus, the contamination becomes my ally: it becomes an "inner reminding factor" which takes me immediately to my inner aims: conscious attention, kindness, generosity, forgiveness, hard work. The fight-flight response *reminds* me to be kind and forgive, it calls me to conscious attention. Thus, instead of making it the enemy (trying to change it, fight it) I have transformed it into my ally and companion in the inner Work. Now there is no more insane fight within. There is cooperation, communication between the centers, harmonious inner working of the human biological instrument for the good of love and for the good of the other. This is unselfish love, objective love. And it does not depend on a feeling, although the feeling of love may be present, but it often is not when the other hurts me. Instead, this kind of objective love depends solely on commitment and practice. Thus it is dependable and consistent, not subject to the tyranny of mood. Mood is like a hunter searching for a deer in the tall grass. If the deer remains still, unmoving, the hunter moves on. Cease identification with what you are not and the hunter has no more ammunition, your suffering is at an end.

Love Is Not A Feeling
(for Smitty)

Love is not a feeling,
it is a commitment etched in stone.
But belief in the feeling sends us reeling
from one failure to another; we end up alone,

broken and cynical. Love is not a feeling,
it is a reliable daily practice.
No matter what I feel, I am not concealing
it, but letting it be. She may be prickly as cactus

and not at all easy on the eye,
the feeling may be disgust,
or let us say she is most lovely
and the feeling is lust; both turn to dust,

still the commitment to practice is steady,
doesn't depend on whether I'm feeling ready.

(Red Hawk)

CHAPTER 19

The Awakening of Conscience— Carrying My Own Cross

Conscience depends upon an understanding of objective suffering.

The least we are asked to be able to do as completed man is to suffer the unpleasant manifestations of others toward ourselves and others without resentment, to take no action against wrongs done us, and to have compassion for those whose nature is more powerful than their being.

(E.J. Gold. *The Joy of Sacrifice*, 99)

> *Teach me to feel another's woe,*
> *To hide the fault I see;*
> *That mercy I to others show,*
> *That mercy show to me.*
> (Alexander Pope. 1688-1744)

The first thing, and the most important thing, to be understood about the path of self observation without judgment or trying to change what is observed is this: the path of self observation is a path of awakening conscience. That is, if I continue to observe myself honestly, long enough, conscience will awaken in me; that is lawful and unavoidable. It is a by-product of honest self observation.

Once conscience has been awakened in the human biological instrument, *woe* is me, because now I will know what conscious (voluntary) suffering really is, and my suffering will take on a whole new dimension that I have never known before. I will deliberately, ruthlessly, slavishly, cruelly go against the still, small *feeling* in me which is conscience (it is misleading to call conscience a "voice" because *it does not speak*; it is a feeling and that is why it suffers). And conscience will never force itself, never be aggressive or insistent or intrusive or violent or critical or judgmental. It will simply pulsate its suffering when it is violated, and it will continue to suffer in feeling-pulsations unless and until I correct my course and make right what and who I have wronged.

Once conscience awakens in me, it suffers every time it is violated. And this suffering is of an order of magnitude, of a new level, that I am not used to. It is suffering which is unbearable and cannot be ignored. It does not demand or condemn, It just suffers, and deeply.

Our practice is to do two things with this suffering: see it and feel it. Period. No need to change anything within: I just see and feel my violation of conscience. This does *not* mean that I do not act externally to right my wrongs. I do. And the quicker I can do that, the sooner the suffering in me is eased. What is left then is the wound which conscience must bear for my behavior. This is known in ancient schools as "the wound of love." In esoteric Christianity, it is called, "carrying one's own cross." This means that I no longer require that God or Guru be my external conscience and suffer my wrongs for me. Now that conscience is awakened in me, I am able to see my mistakes, correct them, suffer them, and trust the internal guidance of conscience. This is trusting reality. This is the recovery of sanity in me.

What is conscience? Masters have suggested that conscience is the direct line of communication with the mind and heart of the Creator; esoteric Christianity has suggested that conscience is the direct link with higher emotional and intellectual centers, which reside at the Source or Creator; my experience appears to validate this view. Other ancient schools have said that conscience is God; I have no experiential reason to doubt this view. Others have said that conscience is the Holy Spirit; still others have suggested that conscience is the awakened soul, or the awakening of self; some in esoteric Christianity have called it "the Ascension of Christ"; and finally, there are those masters who have called the awakening of conscience "the awakening of consciousness."

However you may understand this phenomenon, it is the most real thing a human in the Work will ever undergo. Awakened conscience is the thing in me which can be trusted. Absolutely, always and in everything. Conscience is incapable of lying. It is what the Sufis call the True Friend within; it is the source of real help and guidance on the path. It is the Creator's help in the individual soul's journey towards union with Source.

And such a phenomenon arises lawfully from the persistent, consistent practice of self observation without judgment or trying to change what is observed. I must see and feel my behavior, both within and externally to me. "Wish" and "intention" together can awaken conscience. And eventually, slowly, slowly, what arises in conscience from the combination of "wish" and "intention" is aim. Real aim comes from conscience.

From "aim" I have ally. Now when my inner habitual tendencies arise daily, moment to moment, right alongside them is aim. In fact, at some point, these inner habitual tendencies shift and become inner "reminding factor" to remind me of my aims. Thus, they are transformed from weaknesses, flaws, into faithful servants of my Work; they are brought into my inner *Work circle.** No longer do I fight against them and try to change them, but as they are, they serve my aims and help me. They feed conscience, which allows it to develop, grow, and mature. In the world of the shaman, the ally is a gross, misshapen, terrifying entity with enormous power. Can you see how this is an analogy which applies to one's innermost "flaw" or blind spot? To capture its power and align it with my Work is a feat of power, a "magical pass" in shaman's terms. Self observation is the tool.

In fact, the whole teaching that these things in me which I judge and fight against are "flaws," "weaknesses," is erroneous teaching. Everyone you have ever met without exception has these "flaws." They are given to us as gifts by the Creator. Why? Simple: to assist in the awakening of conscience. Without them, I would not reach the point of valuing what conscience has to offer. I would not develop an inner "wish" or an inner "intention." I would have no force in me for transformation. They are gifts, not flaws. They are where the energy of being is stored, waiting to be released by the simple practice of seeing and feeling their effect upon me and those I love.

Even a mustard seed of conscience—the tiniest, microscopic trace of the mind and heart of our Creator—can become the most powerful force in the human biological instrument. You want miracle? What are you willing to pay to *live in the miraculous*? This mustard seed is the miracle of the Creator's mind and heart placed in the human biological instrument. But you must pay to receive. And voluntary suffering is the only thing we have in us to pay with—it becomes the dearest coin in my purse. So when the

Gospels teach, "A certain *merchant* [man of the Work, rh] sold *all that he had* [his "i's" and their agendas, rh] *in order to purchase a pearl of great price* [conscience, rh]" this is what is meant. Only a desperate man, a man who has suffered "the terror of the situation" for years and years, would be driven to such lengths that he surrendered all that he had to the Creator, in return for this mustard seed, this "pearl of great price." Do you understand?

Conscience is the Creator in me, the direct channel of communication to the mind and heart of the Creator; thus, when I violate conscience, it is the Creator whose suffering I feel—as the direct result of my actions. The Creator willingly and without complaint bears my violations and suffers without complaint. Only when I assume responsibility for my thoughts, emotions, words, and actions does this suffering due to my actions bear fruit. I no longer am comfortable being the cause of my Creator's suffering. Period. Thus, I act at once when out of alignment to keep a clear conscience.

When I *cease to violate conscience* this is a further meaning for "picking up my own cross and carrying it." I no longer ask my Creator to suffer for my sins (the only sin is going against conscience); instead, I become a responsible being. I do as conscience instructs, in order to avoid making my Creator suffer, in order to avoid the terrible, unbearable feeling of that suffering. At that point, I will do anything to avoid the enormity of this feeling, including growing up, including taking responsibility for my own life instead of blaming others and making others suffer my insensitivity, insecurity, and immaturity. At that point, I cease being just a mammal and become a human being.

And when I do bring this suffering upon my Creator, what I feel inside is called "remorse of conscience." This remorse is from on High, it is a gift, and it will transform me. I have seen it. I have experience of it. Remorse is the transformative agent brought by conscience into the human biological instrument.

Now here is a secret, something buried deep into this book so that only those who have paid by reading to this point will find. It is a Work practice which feeds conscience and helps it to grow. Only those souls who have matured to the point of awakened conscience will understand the need for such a practice or feel the value in pursuing it. It is a high-level, mature Work practice, and as such it demands a great deal of me. It produces a whole different level and kind of suffering but its rewards are also of a new order of magnitude; I am rewarded with a different order of relationship among my fellows. A new level of trust results, both within and without. Does such a practice hold interest for you? Here then is how the Work states this practice:

> Bear the unpleasant manifestations of others without complaint or outward show; bear the wrongs done to me without responding in kind. In other words: Do unto others as I would have them do unto me; turn the other cheek.

Perhaps you can see why this is a mature practice, only possible with the help of conscience. It is unthinkable for the ordinary person in life, who could not even imagine why doing such a thing would be of benefit.

But you who have read this far into the book may perhaps intuit the profound implications of this senior Work practice, both for the developing soul and for those with whom I am in relationship. It asks extraordinary things of me: that I sell all that I own. In return, the inner irritation or friction which it produces develops a "pearl of great price." Can you intuit the need and value of such a thing? This provides a new and different level of meaning to the phrase, "carrying my own cross." What is it worth to you? Are you willing to sell your complaining, your gossiping, your negativity, your vengeance and righteous wrath, in order to purchase the services of Conscience, the Guardian Angel?

This practice is difficult for me, but the source of the difficulty may surprise you. It is not friends, colleagues, or even strangers who put this practice to its greatest test in me, though they all do, certainly. No, it is with my wife, whom I love so deeply, and with those closest to me that I have the greatest struggle to hold my tongue and keep my judgments and anger in abeyance. So I have much Work to do with this practice. But I value it deeply and am glad to struggle for it, not against my habits, but for this pearl, for the help which the Guardian Angel provides. Only with its help is there hope for a person. It is my deepest wish and prayer to follow my conscience, always and in everything. This is my aim.

Furthermore, because there is now in me a mustard seed of conscience, not belief systems borrowed from others, but something which is *all my own because I have paid for it*—I wish to sell all that I own to purchase this pearl of great price—now I suffer most intensely, now I suffer in a whole new way and on a whole new level. *And this suffering feeds conscience.* Still there is no need to change anything I observe. Conscience will change everything, and in its own proper and appropriate time and way; I can change nothing and if I try I will make an awful mess of things, just as always.

Tom Kills A Rabbit

Tom was my wife's father. One time
he told me how on his 8th birthday
he got a bow and 6 arrows.
He set up the straw target in his yard

and shot at it for hours until he tired of it,
then set up some smaller, more difficult things,
a can, a piece of paper nailed to a tree,
an old shoe on a log. He was good and

in 3 days or so he tired even of these.
He wanted something more, something lively,
something that would run from him;
he wanted to kill something.

He went into the woods and the first thing
he saw there was a small rabbit frozen in place.
He drew and fired, sent the arrow clean through
the rabbit's body, but it did not die at once;

instead the arrow drove into the ground,
pinning the rabbit there.
Legs churning furiously, it could only spin
wildly around the arrow, blood flowing, its eyes

wild, luminous and hurt.
Tom stood frozen, transfixed with horror and
when he looked up at me his eyes
were hurt like that rabbit's.

He put the bow down, never went back for it.
He was a big man, and that story made him so
for me, how he shot an arrow in the woods
and it pierced his own heart.

(Red Hawk)

CHAPTER 20

Higher Centers

Man, by himself, cannot become a new man; special inner combinations are necessary . . . when such a special matter accumulates in sufficient quantities, it may begin to crystallize, as salt begins to crystallize in water if more than a certain proportion of it is added. When a great deal of fine matter accumulates in a man, there comes a moment when a new body can form and crystallize in him: the "do" of a new octave, a higher octave. This body, often called the astral, can only be formed from this special matter and cannot come into being unconsciously. In ordinary conditions, this matter may be produced in the organism, but is used and thrown out.

(G.I. Gurdjieff. *Views From the Real World*, 202)

Unconditional love, which is conscious love, operates not under mechanical law, but under the laws of conscious behavior. It comes from higher centers and is an act of grace; it is the Creator entering fully, lawfully, and by invitation only, into the human biological instrument. It is the weary Traveler returning home, becoming who it lawfully is: unbounded consciousness without beginning or end. At that point the being makes the lawful bonding-statement: "I am That" or "I and the Father are One." It is a whole different scale and level of love, with an independent set of laws. For example, one law of conscious love is this: Unconditional love engenders the same response in the other. I have seen this law in action in the form of the guru. So I do not speak to you about this law from some book, or borrowed knowledge, or belief system, but from verification by my own personal experience. I work and await the descent of grace in me.

Real love has boundaries. Fear has none. Real relationship operates within very clear and agreed upon boundaries. Failure to honor those boundaries means the relationship cannot endure. Period. End of story. Boundaries in relationship are *not arbitrary* or *secretive*, known only to me. They are mutually agreed upon limits to my behavior, which I willingly enter into because I am committed to the relationship enduring long-term. Period. What takes place in most relationships where two people claim their undying love for one another, is two people operating without agreed upon, mutually acceptable boundaries, in a relationship in which there is no commitment, only what I want, when I want it, and how I want it. This is an infantile emotional level of relationship; it is how babies wish to be treated by their mothers. It is the result of small selfish "i's" having their moment, entering into relationship, and then disappearing. Break down and break-up are the inevitable result of small "i's" in relationship, unconscious beings making mechanical choices and suffering endlessly.

It is not the same when higher centers are activated in the human biological instrument. At that point, unselfish behavior which acts for the good of the other, regardless of the cost to myself, is the result. Conscience is the receiving mechanism for the action of higher centers in me. Once conscience is awakened, then I am at the affect of higher centers voluntarily. By my practice I have issued the invitation which activates their influence in me. Conscience is the manifestation of higher centers in me. It is the law and compels the human being to act in a lawful manner, from basic goodness. This is the nature of the soul and is our birthright. We deserve to be good and to do good. The soul is an angelic being which descends from the angelic world into the human bio-logical instrument to develop the ability to love unconditionally. Earth is the school, a kindergarten for souls, where undeveloped souls are sent to learn. The curriculum is simple but not easy. We are here to learn how to love, without limitations, expectations, or conditions. The means for learning inheres in every human: it is self observation, a single tool for learning. It is all that is ever needed.

To do so, I must collect and store the vibratory energy of incoming impressions, rather than allowing the intellectual-emotional-complex to steal it and use it up in a useless display of endless, repetitive psycho-dramas and mechanical reactions. I must begin to "eat" the vibratory energy of incoming impres-sions. "Sometimes I eat the bear, sometimes the bear eats me," is how the shamanic traditions state this practice. In the mid-twentieth century in New York City, there was a curious man who ran an antique shop. He became something of a legend in spiri-tual circles. He was called Rudi, or Swami Rudrananda. Rudi was an objective eater of vibratory energy impressions and he taught others to do this as well. He worked with the higher centers. He would sit in a room with his students for hours and simply absorb the vibratory energy of incoming impressions, without interfer-ence or identification. He was an objective eater of impressions. This allows the body to activate its higher function, as an "energy transformation instrument." My task is to consciously not interfere with incoming energy, allowing the body to perform its higher functions. If I constantly steal this energy, the body remains fixated on the mammal level, a mere machine.

An objective eater of vibratory energetic impressions is the Work humans were created to do: to help the Creator maintain Its creation and to provide finer substances or food, both for the creation of a higher body within me and to feed higher beings such as the Earth, an angelic being. Look at this from another angle, a simpler analogy, a smaller scale. A carrot enters the body as a very coarse energy which the body cannot use. It must be transformed into a finer, subtler energy in order to be of use. I chew it, breaking it down, mixing it with saliva, then gastric juices, where it is made finer and finer so it can be absorbed through the lining of the stomach and intestines and made into blood. The incoming vibratory energy of impressions is coarse while the Creator exists on a very fine energy, call it love for example, or objective reason, or prana. If I do not interfere with this energy, steal it for selfish psycho-dramas or fantasy, negative emotions, and imagination, then the body is able to assume its higher objective function as a transformational instrument, to feed the Creator, or higher centers. Everything in the universe must eat, this is objective law. The Creator is not exempt.

This path takes courage. Courage doesn't come cheap. Courage is not for heroes, heroes don't need it; courage is for cowards like me. It comes from seeing the horror within so clearly that anything looks better than that. Then I get the courage to go into the unknown, because the known is unacceptable, even unbearable. But the unknown in this case is becoming less mysterious with new discoveries in neural science. Jonah Lehrer writes about some of these discoveries in his *New Yorker* article "The Eureka Hunt." Lehrer cites research done on the prefrontal lobe of the neo-cortex of the brain, in which he reveals, ". . . The prefrontal cortex (the 'top' of the brain) is directly modulating the activity of other areas" (July 28, 2008. 45). Many of these studies center not only on the top of the brain, but on the right hemisphere. This hemisphere is the gateway to the unknown, that part of the brain linked to higher centers. These studies reveal that EEG measurements on subjects register very precise information at the moment when what they call "insight"—and I am calling inspiration— occurs: ". . . The EEG registers a spike of gamma rhythm, which is the highest electrical frequency generated by the brain. Gamma rhythm is thought to come from the 'binding' of neurons, as cells distributed across the cortex draw themselves together into a new network, which is then able to enter consciousness" (43). In other words, the brain is being re-ordered and transformed in the presence of "insight" into wholly new and unknown configurations. This is what meditation and Self Observation do. Lehrer says, "An insight is a fleeting glimpse of the brain's huge store of unknown knowledge. The cortex is sharing one of its secrets" (45).

In the ancient spiritual traditions this is not news. When Lord Sri Krishna instructs Arjuna to place attention ". . . between his eyebrows," he is doing so because masters know that this sustained conscious placement of attention triggers the flow of gamma rhythms in the cortex, those rhythms emanating from the higher centers, and opens it to these higher centers, which are fully operable but we are not plugged in. The result is what they termed "enlightenment." Here's how that works. When I consciously focus the activity of the left hemisphere on finding the body and sensing it, placing attention in the upper part of the prefrontal cortex, this occupies the left hemisphere of the brain so that it cannot continue its random and compulsive searching and sorting of its contents. Now it has found its rightful place in the instrument and slowly, slowly it will come to understand its lawful place. It will come to understand what it can usefully and efficiently do in the operation of the instrument. In some shamanic traditions, this was known as "cleaning the island of the tonal." On one side of the island (brain), all of the various "i's" exist with their multitude of agendas, the asylum, trying to grab the attention. On the other side, the right hemisphere is silent witness, observing without interference. As the multitude on the left cease to be fed on a regular basis, they quiet as well. Now the left hemisphere can assume its higher function, as a passive servant of the right hemisphere which becomes more consciously active, and whose function is to receive input from higher centers. The right hemisphere, once activated consciously, is now a conduit for the unknown, for "insight" and the flow of wisdom. This is another form of meditation, meditation in action. The soul actively meditates upon the body and its functions objectively, without desire or interference and the body passively receives its emanations. The result of such objective meditation is absence of tension in the human biological instrument, diminishment of unnecessary thinking, and gradual cessation of inappropriate emotions. This is what the ancient spiritual traditions have called the "enlightened condition." Now I am a conduit, a "hollow bamboo" as Zen calls it. I am an objective receiver of higher emanations and an objective eater of vibratory energetic impressions. I am an efficient Work-unit in the Creation, maturely and responsibly assuming my lawful place, attuned, in harmony, lawfully aligned with the Creator. This is the highest level of self remembering.

Higher centers are always at work in the body, but their influence is drowned out by the noise of the mind's continuous chatter. I must grow still, "stop the world," in order to receive their influence. By law, I must issue the invitation. Identification masks their influence in me. When I am present to the presence within (yet another level of self remembering), help arrives. Transformation is the result. The brain is re-ordered and the being is transformed.

Calling the Rain Spirit

My daughters and I once drove past a spot
where trees and grass were on fire.
We stopped: 100 degrees, no clouds,
nothing to fight the fire with.
Rain Drop was 5 then. She said she would
call the Rain Spirit   and she did.

Eyes closed she sat there
in the back seat, legs crossed,
and then she fell right over.
She lay totally still.
Little Wind and I watched,
not sure what to do.

A few minutes and she sat up.
A few more and the rain came in sheets
so heavy cars pulled over and stopped.
The fire was put out at once.
I saw it happen. It was child's play.
I do not expect you to believe it;

I only tell you this because I saw
the price we have paid
in trading trust for reason.
Rain Drop knew exactly what to do
and she did it.   I saw it.
I do not expect you to believe it.

(Red Hawk. *Sioux Dog Dance,* 25)

Epilogue

On the journey of the Warrior . . . instead of transcending the suffering of all creatures, we move toward turbulence and doubt however we can. We explore the reality and unpredictability of insecurity and pain, we try not to push it away. If it takes years—if it takes lifetimes—we let it be as it is. At our own pace, without speed or aggression. We move down and down. With us move millions of others, our companions in awakening from fear. (Pema Chödrön)

In order to see clearly, with sensitivity and real objectivity, it is imperative that one find a way to take absolutely no position in relationship to thought, feeling and experience. It is a very difficult thing to do. In spite of that, it must be done; and indeed, the discovery of the ability to take no position in relationship to thought, feeling and experience is the very ground of the Enlightened perspective . . . One has to somehow find a way through contemplation and meditation to take no position in order to be able to perceive the Real . . . Finally, one has to ask oneself: What position am I taking and to what degree am I truly able to take no position in relationship to what I'm perceiving? This kind of meditation must be sustained. It's not something that can be done just once and then left. (Andrew Cohen. "The Paradox of the Fully Awakened Condition." *What Is Enlightenment?* 2:1 [January 1993]. 6-7)

You are not really tired of being afraid or you would drop it. Somewhere you don't want to let go of it, you are clinging to it. You can't change yourself, nothing can change you: no Primal Therapy, or Encounter groups—nothing. All that can happen is that you can come to accept yourself. Even God can't change you. Otherwise why did he make you like this, and why couldn't he change you if you were not right? And if he did change you then you wouldn't be who you are. He made you the only way it was possible to make you. You think you are ugly, then be ugly. You don't like your body, you don't like your mind—they are you, accept them . . .

And it is the ego that wants to change, become radiant, enlightened, unique. No one loves themselves. And this is the whole beautiful attitude of the religious man—that nothing can be changed, so eat well, live, enjoy. He doesn't waste energy fighting against himself. Nothing is wrong but a wrong attitude. You are trying to square the circle—it can't be done; if it could, it would no longer be a circle. (Osho Rajneesh. Pre-Darshan Notes. Poona, India: June 26, 1975)

Glossary of Terms

Aim: the result of the combined forces of Intention (from the intellectual center) and Wish (from the emotional center); Real Aim comes from Conscience and is the beginning of Will (see also: **Intention, Will**)

Attention: the act of focusing the mind, feelings, and Being on an object or process; the Being is Attention in a human body; Consciousness (see also: **Being**).

Basic Goodness: the true Being-nature unencumbered by ego-interference; the Being instructed and guided by Conscience (suggested by Chögyam Trungpa Rinpoche).

Being: called variously Soul, Atman, Spirit; it is Attention or Consciousness, undeveloped in ordinary life, developed only through special effort, Conscious effort (see also: **Attention**).

Blind Spot: known variously as Chief Feature, Cramp, Petty Tyrant, Contamination, Chief Fault, or Chief Flaw; the Wizard behind the screen; the core feature around which the psycho-emotional structure or ego is built. It is obvious to everyone but oneself, to whom no amount of evidence can convince me of its centrality.

Buffers: a system whose function is to protect the ego-structure and prevent me from seeing myself as I am; to prevent me from seeing the contradictions of various small "i's" in me; composed of many things, among which are blame, justification, self impor-tance, and self pity.

Centers: some systems might call these Chakras, points of energy transformation in the body; here we consider mainly 4 centers: intellectual (head-brain), emotional (solar plexus-heart center), instinctive (navel), and moving (base of the spine). The Work also teaches of two higher intellectual and emotional centers, which exist outside of, but connected to and accessible by, the body.

Conscience: the organic link in the Human Biological Instrument to the Mind and Heart of the Creator; the source of Real Will (see also: **Will**). Also called by some Holy Spirit and by others Guardian Angel.

Consciousness: The elemental life force or intelligence in all sentient beings; the 'I Am' sense of being or presence; the sense that I exist; free attention without the interference of ego. In humans, it is possible through conscious effort to develop and mature this force to the level of the Creator; self observation is one means of doing this.

Contamination: identification, with the body and its functions and conditioning, or with external objects and people; the Blind Spot (see also: **Blind Spot**); the programs placed into the body's energy-centers by those well-meaning (or otherwise) but ignorant beings who influenced us in childhood: these programs define, limit and circumscribe the self, life, and the world, they control how and what we see and feel.

Corridor of Madness: The point in the process of self observation when the buffer system is erased, the blind spot is fully revealed, resistance to Work is fierce, and inner Armageddon ensues. The only hope for my Work to survive is full reliance on Guru, Dharma, Sangha, and practice. A shift in context must occur here (see chapter 17).

Creator: Who knows? Not me. Possibly I.

Ego: the entire psycho-emotional structure, housed not only in the intellectual-emotional-complex, but also in moving center as various postures and movements.

Honest Body: A consciously relaxed body, especially in moments of stress; a body without the unnecessary tensions of identification.

Human Biological Instrument: the human body viewed from a more Objective viewpoint.

Identification: I-am-that; the belief that I am only the body or the body's processes or functions, or anything other than Attention.

Intention: From the intellectual center, although it can be deeper, possibly from the Being; when it is combined with Wish from emotional center, it can be the beginning of Will (see also: **Wish, Will**).

Labyrinth: another name for the intellectual-emotional-complex.

Mechanical: driven by habit; automatic pilot; unconscious; unaware.

Negative Emotion: all fear-based emotions other than those related to present-danger to the organism; those emotions which are not love.

Objective: the view of an object or process without the interference of ego, its beliefs, opinions, judgments, likes and dislikes, that is: without identification with the object or process (see also: **identification, ego**)

Sensation: the movement of energy in the body, as revealed by Attention as well as the input of the 5 senses.

Soul: (see Being).

Voluntary Suffering: different from the ordinary suffering of humanity which is due to the action of habit and belief systems, expectations and desire; the result of the Conscious Intention to observe myself honestly, without judgment or trying to change what is observed; unlike ordinary mechanical suffering, Voluntary Suffering has the power to transform the Being.

Will: the Conscious focus of intellectual, emotional, and instinctive-moving centers simultaneously upon an object, action, direction, or process; the ability to direct the Attention (see also: **Wish, Aim**).

Will of Attention: The fundamental, minimal ability to consciously direct the attention onto an object or inner process, even in the grip of identification, and when no other action is possible; the ability to see myself as I am in the midst of my daily life.

Wish: from emotional center, it can be deeper, possibly from Being; it is the result of Voluntary Suffering and is the first cry for help, when I see the need for inner change (see also: **Aim, Intention, Will**).

Work: (also Practical Work On Self): Conscious, intentional inner labor to observe myself as I am, without judgment or trying to change what is observed; remembering myself in the midst of my daily life; voluntary suffering as a result of observing myself as I am, without buffers, lying, blaming, or justifying.

Work Circle: (or Inner Work Circle): The inner, non-judgmental space created by non-identification with what is observed, which allows what arises within me to do so without interference; those small inner "i's" and groups of "i's" which have bonded together to support inner Work; the connection of mind and body via sensation which allows the harmonious working of centers.

References

Peter Brook. "The Secret Dimension." In: *Gurdjieff: Essays and Reflections on the Man and His Teaching.* Ed. Needleman, Jacob and George Baker. Continuum: New York, 1996.

Buddha. *Dhammapada.* Tr. Thomas Byrom. New York: Viking Press, 1976.

de Salzmann, Michel. *Material for Thought* 14. San Francisco: Far West Editions, 1995.

Gold, E.J. *The Joy of Sacrifice: Secrets of the Sufi Way.* Prescott, Arizona: Hohm Press, 1978.

Gurdjieff, G.I. *Views From the Real World.* New York: Penguin Books, 1973.

Lannes, Henriette. *Inside A Question.* London: Paul H. Crompton. Ltd., 2002.

Lao Tsu. *Tao Te Ching.* Translated by Gia-fu Feng. New York: Viking, 1972. Sutra 33.

Lozowick, Lee. *Feast or Famine: Teachings on Mind and Emotions.* Prescott, Arizona: Hohm Press, 2008.

Osho. *The Dhammapada: The Way of the Buddha.* Portland, Ore: Rebel Publishing House, n.d.

Ouspensky, P.D. *The Fourth Way.* New York: Vintage Books, 1957.

Red Hawk. *The Art of Dying.* Prescott, Arizona: Hohm Press, 1999.

Red Hawk. *The Sioux Dog Dance.* Cleveland: Cleveland State University Press, 1991.

Red Hawk. *The Way of Power.* Prescott, Arizona: Hohm Press, 1996.

Red Hawk. *Wreckage With A Beating Heart.* Prescott, Arizona: Hohm Press, 2005.

Young, Mary. *As It Is.* Prescott, Arizona: Hohm Press, 2000.

About the Author

Red Hawk was the Hodder Fellow at Princeton University and currently teaches at the University of Arkansas at Monticello. His other books are: *Journey of the Medicine Man* (August House); *The Sioux Dog Dance* (Cleveland State University); *The Way of Power* (Hohm Press, 1996); *The Art of Dying* (Hohm Press, 1999); and *Wreckage With a Beating Heart* (Hohm Press, 2005). He has published in such magazines as *The Atlantic*, *Poetry*, and *Kenyon Review*, and has given readings with Allen Ginsberg (1994), Rita Dove (1995), Miller Williams (1996), Tess Gallagher (1996), and Coleman Barks (2005), and more than seventy solo-readings in the United States. Red Hawk is available for readings, lectures, and workshops. He may be contacted at 824 N. Hyatt, Monticello, AR, 71655; or via e-mail at: moorer@uamont.edu

Hohm Press
P.O. Box 2501
Prescott, AZ 86302
800-381-2700
Visit our website at www.hohmpress.com